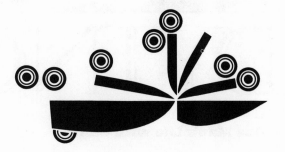

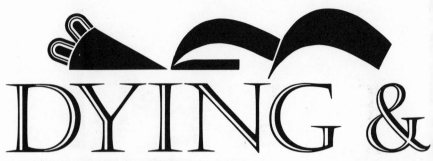

DYING &

One Man's Life with Cancer

by Kenneth A. Shapiro

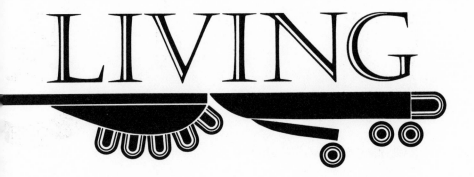

LIVING

 University of Texas Press, Austin

First Edition, 1985

Book design and typographic ornamentation
by George Lenox

Requests for permission to reproduce material
from this work should be sent to Permissions,
University of Texas Press, Box 7819, Austin, Texas 78713.

LIBRARY OF CONGRESS
CATALOGING IN PUBLICATION DATA

Shapiro, Kenneth A. (Kenneth Allen), 1942–
  Dying & living.

  1. Shapiro, Kenneth A. (Kenneth Allen), 1942–
2. Cancer—Patients—United States—Biography. I. Title.
[DNLM: 1. Medical Oncology—personal narratives.
2. Patient Compliance—personal narratives.
QZ 200 S5285d]
RC265.6.S53A33   1985   362.1'96994 [B]   84-25743
ISBN 0-292-70380-5

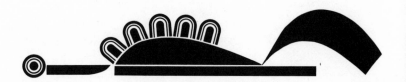

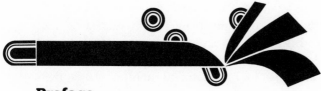

Preface

Writing a book of any sort is quite an accomplishment. Aside from strictly technical books, there is no way that a great deal of what the author is doesn't go into the finished product. In my case, more than can be described has gone into this book. It was written to give me an avenue of expression that was no longer available elsewhere for various reasons. Since late March 1978, when I started on it, writing has been a great release for me, and I hope the book brings some comfort to others, either individuals with cancer or their family and friends, knowing that others have been there before. Perhaps, learning from my experiences, they can avoid some of the quagmires that I have fallen into. I have certainly done many things right but just as certainly I have done other things wrong. I have taken upon myself more of the therapeutic decision-making responsibilities than most physicians are accustomed to, but I have more at stake than anyone else and will not permit others to make decisions of this magnitude for me. Sometimes I have created bigger problems than were necessary that not only could have but should have been avoided. In short, I hope others can learn from my successes and my failures.

This book is not meant to hurt or embarrass any person, organization, or institution. It is simply the way I see what has happened to me and what I have experienced as an individual who has cancer and is doing his best to fight it and anything else that gets in the way of the fight. In retrospect, I hope to show that any disease, but especially cancer, is more than a physical disease destroying more than the physical body. It can, perhaps worst of all, destroy not only the patient's but also the family's emotional as well as mental stability and financial security. As an example, let me relate a short story about a person who was diagnosed as having terminal cancer but couldn't afford the treatments he needed over and above the insurance benefits. He sold his house and bought a trailer, which he and his family lived in while he traveled back and forth for his treatment. In his case it worked and he is alive today. However, what would have happened if it hadn't worked? Then his wife and family would have been left living in a trailer someplace with no roots and financially ruined. What then? There are certain things that you can control and you must know in your own mind beforehand how far it is that you are willing to go and how much you are willing to sacrifice in order to continue the fight. If that sounds like I am saying there is a price for life, under certain circumstances, that is exactly what I am saying, especially if the patient is the main breadwinner of the family. However, in those circumstances only that individual can make the decisions as to where the parameters that cannot be crossed lie. I think it important to point out that this book is being written from the point of view of a person who not only has cancer and has been diagnosed as being terminal but also is the primary wage earner of the family and is worried about the impact his death would have upon his family. How would they be able to survive emotionally and financially? It is a very different situation when the person with the disease is not the major provider because in that case all that is financially sacrificed often can be built up again. When you bear the financial responsibility for the family you naturally want them to be able to survive at a certain economic level if you should die. Therefore, unless you have a guarantee of success, can you in good conscience sacrifice everything on a gamble when the odds are stacked incredibly against you?

People tend to shudder at the word *cancer*, but when it is   **9**
applied to themselves, there is outright fear and terror. There
is no doubt that cancer can be a killer, physically, emotionally,
financially. I say can be, not must be. Advances are being
made; fascinating and, one hopes, fruitful research is being
done. Cures are not here yet for all cancers but they are closer,
and sooner or later they will be realities. However, we do not
have to help cancer cause its destruction. If you happen to
have cancer you owe it to yourself to fight, to give yourself the
very best chance you can. You owe it to yourself not to let cancer beat you unnecessarily. You owe it to yourself to be fighting mentally and supporting the physical struggle going on.
The mental support you give yourself is equally as important
as the physical support your physicians are trying to give
you. It is a well-documented fact that those people who have
the mental tenacity to fight do better than those who just quit
as soon as they are told of their cancer. No matter what course
you choose to follow, the fight is not an easy one; however,
the only requirement in any course of action you might take is
that you truly believe in what you are doing. Some of the
therapies are more difficult than others. Some are almost de-
humanizing, but if you truly believe in what you are doing
you have a better chance of beating the cancer than if you are
just a body receiving a drug. I sometimes wonder if the people
who are recommending this drug or that drug would subject
their bodies to the therapy they are recommending. Of course
they will probably say they would but when it really came
down to the nitty-gritty I wonder what they would do. But
they are not the ones taking the treatments, you are, and you
are the one who must remain in control; you are the one who
must make your own decisions and make sure you remain the
central figure and not just a body in a drug program. That is
one of the things this book is about.

I want to say thanks to some of the people who have helped
me a great deal in my fight against cancer and in making this
book become a reality. First of all, I want to thank the people
of Champion Products, Inc., in Rochester, New York. They

10   have been more than my former employers. I have been retired for over two years now and they continue to stand by
me every step of the way. They remember me and care about
what happens to me. Every time something goes wrong they
are always there doing whatever they can to help. Sometimes
that means just a card or flowers or a phone call; sometimes
that means much more and they have been there each and
every time. The net result of this has always been a tremendous spur for me to fight on and regain my strength and
some semblance of health. In particular I want to single out
three individuals who have gone more than out of their way
to help me. First is Dick Geisler, past president and chairman
of the board of Champion, who himself died of cancer in June
of 1984. He made certain that everything that could be done
for me was done plus more. He was a good man. Next is
Roger Vallercorse, who has fought my battles for me with the
insurance companies. Without him I wouldn't have had a
chance in hell of winning at all with them. He has gone out on
a limb for me time and again. He made my decision to retire
as bearable as one could and made sure that no matter what I
decided not only he and Mr. Geisler but all of Champion
would stand with me and make the decision work. Finally,
there is Harold Lipson. For eighteen years he has been there
for me, helping, guiding, giving me the moral support I
needed. He has been an advisor, but especially a friend. He
has been a force in many of my successes and a large part in
my fight against cancer. He has supported and encouraged me
in my decisions and has never forgotten me. He would call to
see how things were going after I retired, especially when
things weren't going well. His support has been invaluable.
He has never forgotten, and for those who don't understand
what that means, I don't think there is a higher compliment
that can be said in my particular situation. Without the support of Champion and these three men in particular, I can
catagorically say that I would not be alive today. How can you
say thanks for that, other than to just say, THANKS.
    Many doctors have been involved with my case but there
are several who continue to be active now as well as in the

past not only as doctors but as friends and advisors as well. The doctors names used here and throughout the book are fictitious but they know who they are, and I want to thank each of them. Dr. Johnson, our family doctor and godfather to my son, found the original basal cell and continues to consult on my case and watches out for new and interesting developments that might have some bearing on me. Dr. Wesley, another family friend, diagnosed and treated the original basal cell and also continues to look out for new and different approaches to treating melanoma that might help me. Dr. Kenyon pulled me out of the first C-Parvum treatment and has been with me ever since through all the treatments and all the hard times, not only as a doctor but also as a friend and an advisor and seems to have a sixth sense about what I have been going through. He is now devoting full time to research. It is a shame he has been lost to the patients. However, with his intelligence and intuition about cancer, perhaps he will be the biggest help of all in contributing to finding the causes of cancer. My two main doctors in Houston, Dr. Fredericks and Dr. Alberts, have never given up. No matter what the situation has been, they have always been there saying we could do this or that or whatever. They have supported me medically but also emotionally and it has been greatly appreciated. Dr. Diaz, who was willing to take a chance when the big names said no and with his surgical skill and knowledge made it pay off, is continuing to look into several therapies that have never been tried before but look promising. Dr. Abrams, not only a great doctor but also a great human being and a friend, has operated on me so many times he probably knows my body better than his own. He knew what he was doing and he knew when it was time to send me to someone else who knew more. His judgment has been impeccable. He was responsible for sending me to M. D. Anderson Hospital and has continued to work with my doctors there to make sure that everything that could be done is done. He has stood beside me through everything. When I needed medical advice he has always been available and when he didn't know the answer he found out. He has trusted my judgment almost as

12   much as I have trusted his. Together we have made it to this point, but without him there wouldn't be any "this point" at all. He not only has called me when I have been in the hospital out of town but also checks with my family to make sure they are doing well too. He cares, and he has treated me not so much as a patient but as a human being who has not only a physical problem but emotions that go along with it. He truly is the personification of what a doctor should be.

I want to thank Jean Busfield, who has helped and encouraged me with this book. Her daughter, Terry Schmit, was most helpful in putting the manuscript in order. A big thanks to all my friends and relatives who have helped in many ways, but especially during the times I have been in the hospital and my wife desperately needed their help and support and they gave it. Finally, I want to thank the staff of the University of Texas Press, as well as its faculty advisory committee, for taking a chance and publishing this book. They have offered advice, support, and encouragement to a totally unknown author. I want to especially thank them for giving me the opportunity to help others who might read this book and find some comfort and help from it.

Kenneth A. Shapiro
September 1984

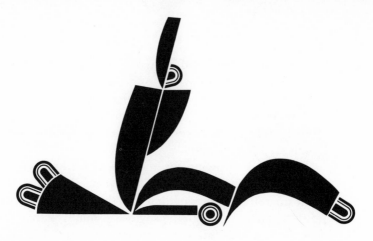

Chapter 1

I was born in New York in 1942. My earliest memories are those of moving from one house on Long Island to the house that I grew up in, also on Long Island. I was four years old at the time and we lived right across the street from the elementary school where I went from kindergarten through the eighth grade. I was a normal, perhaps average child, although I was always getting into trouble of one sort or another. If there was a fight I was usually involved in some fashion. If anyone ever got caught with a yo-yo or a water pistol in school, it was sure to be me. Whenever there was any trouble at all, the principal would stand at the front door and single out the five or six troublemakers and say, "Shapiro, to my office." Usually he was right. I hated school until my junior year in high school. I was much more interested in sports than academics, until I learned that you need to be competent in both in order to be able to participate in athletics. At first I was only interested in baseball, and then it was baseball and basketball, and finally it was exclusively basketball. I ran track and cross-country but only to stay in shape for basketball. I lettered in all of these sports on the varsity level and in my senior year I was the captain of the basketball team. I had kept my grades just high enough to be eligible to participate in sports. I was a very good athlete, too, but more because I was willing to work hard than because of any great amount of natural ability. I used to practice basketball during the off-season almost three hours a day, every day, even if it meant practicing by myself, which often was the case. During my junior year I finally decided to buckle down and start to get the grades that I should have been getting and it paid off. I went to college and eventually graduated with a degree in business administration.

While I was growing up my parents worked very hard to provide our family with the things we needed. My father was a salesman for a company that sold dry cleaning supplies and he always made enough to provide the family with everything that we needed, but we were certainly not rich—it was a struggle. At times my mother worked in a bank but for the most part she was a housewife and mother. My father died of cancer at the age of 64, barely eight weeks before my son, his only grandchild, was born. He would have loved to have seen him just once before he died. I wish that he were still alive, not only so that he could see his grandson, but so I could tell him how much I appreciated all the things that he and my mother did for us and all of the sacrifices that they made for my brother and me. I especially wish that he were still alive so that I could tell him before he died that I loved him very much.

In June of 1960, I entered C. W. Post College, in Greenville, New York, but I really wasn't very happy there because I thought I was going to be the next great college basketball star and I wanted to be at a basketball powerhouse school. The following January, I transferred to Bradley University in Illinois, which at the time was the number-two basketball school in the country. Being a transfer student I had to sit out for a year but I did practice with the team during that time and I loved every minute of it. However, right before I became eligible I caught pneumonia and had to leave school. I also realized that although I was a good basketball player I wasn't a great basketball player and would never be the star that I had dreamed I would be when I went out there. I left Bradley and after recovering from the pneumonia I joined the army. At least I had the good sense to realize that I wasn't going anywhere doing what I was doing, so I might as well get the mili-

tary service out of the way, and, as things turned out, it was a great move.

When I informed my parents that I had joined the army, they were, to put it mildly, less than enthusiastic. They tried everything to stop me, including calling the enlistment officer to persuade him to turn me down. However, I was eighteen and I knew they couldn't stop me. Nothing worked and on March 1, 1962, I left at 5:00 A.M. in order to sign the final papers and leave for Fort Dix and basic training that same day. As I was leaving, my mother confronted me with, "If you leave and join the army, don't ever return to this house." I was sorry she felt that way, but if that's what she really wanted then I would have to accept it. Eventually, she calmed down and a truce was reached. However, even if it hadn't been, I felt that at eighteen it was time for me to start taking responsibility for my own actions. I needed to start making my own decisions—to accept responsibility if I made the wrong ones and to pat myself on the back if I made the right ones. My attitude has been the same ever since.

Except for a four-month tour of duty in Thailand, I spent most of my time in the army playing basketball in Hawaii. I was actually assigned to an army aviation unit, but because I was away so much playing basketball on one team or another I was put in charge of an athletic office for the last twenty months of service. I actually enjoyed the time in Thailand more than anything else that I did in the service. It was truly an education. About ten of us were stationed way up-country in a little town called Roi Et. Although there were none of the conveniences that we have come to expect, such as plumbing and electricity, I really enjoyed it. It was a tremendous experience to live among people who don't have all the luxuries that we have. I learned more about life there than any place I had been up to that point in my life. We lived in tents in a clearing in the jungle. There were water buffalo all over the place and among some of the other local wildlife were cobras, scorpions, tarantulas, red ants that thought of humans as a delicacy, and a tiny green snake about the size of a worm that is sup-

posedly one of the world's most deadly snakes and likes to hide in the trees where it is virtually invisible. Since there wasn't any running water to take a shower we had to improvise. It was the rainy season for most of the time that we were over there and it rained almost like clockwork at 1:00 P.M. When it rained it really poured and we simply took off our clothes, got a bar of soap, and showered right then and there. I'm really not sure what we were doing there. We were part of a much larger, multinational war games unit that I guess was supposed to be a show of force to the communists, who were beginning to be a big problem in Viet Nam at the time.

After I was discharged from the army in 1965, I returned to C. W. Post College on a basketball scholarship. I knew by then that my future was not in basketball, but it was a way of paying for my college education. I got another scholarship for running the intramural program for the college, and I worked as a waiter on weekends at a very nice local restaurant. I hit the books extra hard to make sure I kept a good grade-point average and graduated in January of 1967. While at Post I met Lynne. I was working in the girls' cafeteria at the time and I just went over and sat down and introduced myself to her one day. She was actually a year ahead of me but that was because I had missed some school while I was in the army. We hit it off fairly well and started dating but then she got engaged to someone else and we didn't see each other for about seven months. She graduated and started teaching out on Long Island. I didn't see her again until just before I graduated in 1967. I told her I would write to her and let her know where I was going to be as soon as I knew. With the army behind me and my degree in my pocket, I was ready to tackle the world. I was hired right out of college by Champion Knitwear, Inc. (the company name at that time). Champion is a very fine athletic and resale knitwear company and has through the years been extraordinarily good to me. My career with Champion was the first and last full-time job that I ever anticipated having.

Champion sent me to Lansing, Michigan, where I became the area sales representative. I let Lynne know where I was and several months later I got a letter from her saying that she

was no longer engaged. On a return trip to New York I called **17**
her and we started dating again. In July 1968 we were married
and she got a job teaching school in Lansing. She was doing
some modeling also, mainly because it made her feel good to
keep a little active in the glamourous part of her life. She
probably could have been one of the top fashion models in
the country if she had pursued modeling rather than teaching. We lived in several apartments before building our own
house. The house was something that I really wanted but not
something that Lynne really wanted. I think that it represented
too much of a commitment to her. However, because of the
tax advantages, we decided to go ahead with it and I really
had a great time helping to design the house and watching it
go up each step of the way. It's a fairly modern house on a
wooded lot on a cul-de-sac in East Lansing. Even though she
doesn't like to admit it, I think Lynne has finally decided to
like the house too. On March 24, 1976, the greatest thing that
has ever happened to me occurred. Our son, Jared, was born.
I wanted a child very badly but again Lynne really didn't because that was a commitment that she didn't want to make.
However, I don't think there is anything in the world she
would rather have now than our son.

After graduating from college and going to work for Champion, I was doing very well and enjoying what I was doing.
At first I was selling almost exclusively to the high school and
junior high market. After about six years I was given the college market, too, and I started calling on Michigan State, the
University of Michigan, and all the college accounts in the territory that I had. I really enjoyed that. I was able to be home
almost every night and the people I was dealing with were
very nice. As a matter of fact, some of the people who started
out as customers have become some of my very closest friends.
I was working my way up in the sense that the more I developed the territory the more I sold, and the more I sold the
more I made. As this developed, it reached the point where I
had Champion bring another man into the territory. That
made three of us in Michigan and we have been close friends
ever since that time. All during this time Lynne was also

working and developing a very fine reputation as an excellent teacher. She took six weeks off when Jared was born and then returned to work. Nothing was further from my mind than the possibility that at age 35 I would be struck with cancer.

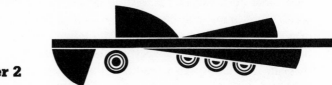

Chapter 2

I had never been sick with anything even remotely serious other than the pneumonia I had when I left Bradley. In April of 1977 I had a sore throat that seemed to persist, so I went to the doctor. In the past when this happened, he would look at it and give me a prescription for some antibiotics, and within twenty-four hours I was feeling fine again. That's exactly what happened this time, too, with one difference. During the course of the examination, Dr. Johnson, our family physician, good friend, and my son's godfather, noticed that a light spot on my forehead had changed slightly in color. He literally took me by the hand and marched me across the hall into another doctor's office. Dr. Wesley, who is also a friend, is a dermatologist. Suddenly I had three physicians crowding around, looking at this spot, and I still had no idea what was going on. Dr. Wesley said that he couldn't tell for sure but that it might be a basal cell carcinoma. He went on to explain that this was a form of skin cancer and nothing to get excited about, as long as it was taken care of. They decided that it should be excised for a biopsy immediately, which they did.

The results came back confirming that it was indeed a basal cell. Dr. Wesley again explained that this was really nothing to be concerned about. The form of treatment that he decided on was one in which a cream would be used that would burn the basal cell out and leave no detectable scar. After several weeks of this treatment, Dr. Wesley, upon examining the area again, said that it still didn't feel right, although it felt different than before. He wanted to repeat the biopsy and recheck the results against the first one. This time the results were that it

was still a basal cell but a more difficult one to treat than before. Dr. Wesley explained that the best way to treat this type was to cut it out. I was referred to Dr. Abrams, a plastic surgeon who specializes in head and neck surgery, especially head and neck *cancer* surgery. I have learned a great deal about Dr. Abrams over the past few years. We have seen each other often enough, usually in the operating room. We once were joking around in the operating room that we must stop meeting like this. After examining me and consulting with Dr. Wesley, Dr. Abrams agreed that the best course of action was to remove it surgically, which he did several weeks later.

Everything went well until June 9, when I went to Dr. Abrams' office for a follow-up after the removal of all the stitches. I very casually asked about a spot on the back of my left shoulder. I thought that Dr. Abrams was going to have a coronary. He immediately scheduled a biopsy in the hospital and within an hour I was lying on a stretcher waiting to be taken into the operating room. I didn't have time to notify anyone, not even Lynne, who was teaching at school. Dr. Abrams explained to me that until the biopsy results were in he couldn't be sure, but he was afraid I had a very serious problem, one that must be taken care of immediately. He suspected that it was a malignant melanoma, and he explained to me what that meant. It still didn't mean a great deal to me, because I had never even heard of a malignant melanoma. After the biopsy, which was on a Thursday, Dr. Abrams said that I should call him late Friday afternoon for the results. After I left the hospital I went right to the library to find out what a malignant melanoma was. I found out. I learned that melanoma was the only fatal form of skin cancer, that it was one of the most deadly forms of cancer known, and that the only sure thing about it was its total unpredictability. I wasn't quite sure how to tell Lynne what was happening. I wasn't quite sure myself what was happening so how could I tell someone else. After all, what could I say, "Hi, dear, how was your day, mine was just fine. Oh, by the way I spent the afternoon in the hospital and found out that I might have a fatal form of cancer." What I did tell her was that during the course of his examination Dr.

Abrams looked at a spot that I had pointed out to him and decided that it looked suspicious enough to warrant a biopsy. Since he was going to be in the hospital that afternoon anyway, he thought it would be a good idea to do it right then, and that I was to call him the following afternoon to get the results. I tried to leave it at that. However, Lynne wanted to know what Dr. Abrams thought it was and I told her. Fortunately, she didn't have any more of an idea of what a melanoma was than I had had; however, she knew that it didn't sound very good. I told her that we wouldn't know for sure until the results were in the next day and that it didn't make any sense to worry about it until then, if at all.

By the time I got home on Friday, Dr. Abrams had already called and left word that he wanted to see me at once. I went to his office along with Lynne and Jared. Dr. Abrams explained that the biopsy showed that it was indeed quite serious and should be taken care of immediately. He said that the biopsy showed it to be a malignant melanoma level III. He said that he had taken the liberty of calling the National Cancer Research Institute (NCRI) in Washington, D.C., to check their recommendations, and they had confirmed his opinion. He explained the procedure, saying there would be skin grafts involved and that, although it would not be a pleasant experience, the surgery itself was not of a life-or-death nature. I decided that since things were happening so fast I would not tell anyone else in my family. My mother and some of my family lived in New York, my brother in Winnipeg, Canada, some cousins and an aunt in Kentucky, others in California; it would just be too cumbersome for anyone to have to drop whatever it was they were doing to come to Lansing—and do what? I really didn't see any need for anyone to come at that time. I knew that my mother, as well intentioned as she is, would have insisted that I go to one of the larger East Coast cancer centers to get a second opinion. Under other circumstances that would probably have been a good idea, but in this case time was very important. Dr. Abrams was leaving the country for two months shortly and I really wanted him to do the surgery. With Dr. Johnson, Dr. Wesley, and the NCRI all concurring on the course of action to take, I felt that the decision I made was the best one. I have never regretted that decision. On Monday, June 13, 1977, I entered the hospital and on Tuesday the surgery was performed.

I did try to reach my brother, who was en route from Winnipeg to Philadelphia for a conference and from there to New York to visit our mother. I called him at his conference, but I missed him. He had already left for New York. I hesitated telling him while he was with Mom, but, sensitive to the situation, he did not indicate to her that anything was at all wrong. He asked me to stick around the house for awhile and said he would call me back. He immediately went to the library (it must run in the family) and then called me. Even though he is a psychologist, he wasn't sure what a malignant melanoma was either, so he looked it up and wasn't pleased with what he found out. When he called he was obviously shaken and wanted to know more of the details. He wanted to be certain that I was doing the right thing. I assured him that I was and I suggested that he call Lynne on Tuesday night at home and she would let him know how everything went. Although upset, he wished me luck and told me that if we needed him he would fly out immediately. Just in case anything went wrong I thought it best that he know what was going on and that he stay with Mom.

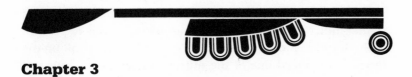

Chapter 3

On Monday the thirteenth I checked into the hospital; after being shown to my room, I promptly left to make some calls on a few customers that I had to see. I told Dr. Abrams I was going to do that and he agreed, saying he would try to cover for me with the hospital staff. Anyway, I felt they could do all the tests they needed in the evening. There were things I had to get done that were my responsibility and that I couldn't do sitting around a hospital room, accomplishing nothing at all other than worrying about what was to happen the following day. The hospital personnel were angry with me but were to learn that this was not going to be the last time that I did something like that. They also have ways of getting even, too. It seemed that they ran not only all of the necessary tests but also most of the unnecessary tests in existence that night.

On Tuesday several close friends came to spend some time with me and to wish me luck. Their support was especially helpful to Lynne, and I appreciated their concern for both of us. Since I wasn't scheduled for surgery until late in the afternoon, I advised Lynne not to take the day off from work. I felt it would be better for her to keep some sense of normality in her day. She arrived at about three-thirty. Jared was home with the babysitter. I had been given a shot to relax me about a half-hour before she got there. At four o'clock the surgical nurses came to take me down for the surgery. The last thing that I remember is getting the sodium pentothol and going right out. I woke up in the recovery room only briefly, was taken back to my room, was given something for the pain, and then slept until morning. When I awoke, breakfast arrived. I wasn't very hungry. I was told not to use my left arm because of the surgery and the possibility of disrupting the skin grafts. I had an I.V. tube in my right arm and it was taped to a board that immobilized my right hand. This being the case, I was wondering what I was supposed to do with the breakfast that was sitting in front of me. The I.V. seemed rather ludicrous, since the only reason I had it was to prevent dehydration, and now that I was awake I could drink on my own. I convinced one of the nurses to take the I.V. out and remove the board along with it. I had told her that if she didn't, I would.

Dr. Abrams arrived a little later and said that I had come through the operation just fine. I couldn't tell what had been done because it was all on the back part of my left shoulder. I not only couldn't see it but it was so numb I couldn't feel it either. However, I was acutely aware of pain elsewhere. Dr. Abrams told me that he had taken the skin for the graft from

the upper part of my buttock. That's where the most graftable   **23**
skin is, due to the fact that it has never been exposed to the
sun and the elements. He said it would be uncomfortable for
a while, but it would heal eventually and be just as good as
new. He was right of course, but to this day the donor site still
looks very much like the patch on the back pocket of a pair of
Levi jeans. For me it also gave new meaning to the phrase
"pain in the butt." The one thing that Dr. Abrams didn't tell
me was that while it was healing it wouldn't be just uncomfortable, it would be as painful as hell. Everything that would
touch the area would stick to it and cause a lot of pain and
then getting it off be even worse. (I have learned in my experiences with the medical profession how to interpret some of
the phrases, such as a "little discomfort": that means PAIN
and more than just a little.) The burn unit was in charge of the
graft donor site and for certain periods during the day they
would have me lying on my stomach completely naked while
they had a special light shining on the donor site to promote
the healing process. Since I had to be totally naked for this
process, my room was closed off and a sign put up that said,
All visitors for Ken Shapiro please report to the nurses' station. Unfortunately, the first time this happened some friends were
on their way to see me and when they saw this sign they
thought I had died.

I remained in the hospital for twelve days after this operation and while I was still there my brother stopped in on his
way back to Winnipeg. I think he was reassured when he had
a chance to see me and talk with me. He could see for himself
that I wasn't withering away and was not about to pack it in
and call it quits. We discussed the entire situation and we decided that at least for the time being it would serve no purpose at all to tell Mom. I could tell her at a later date when I
had more information as to what the prognosis was and what
the future was going to hold for me. Since he hadn't seen
Jared since he was born, he stayed for a few days to visit, not
only me but also Lynne and Jared. He stayed for a few days,
then returned home feeling much better about the situation.
After ten days at home, I was allowed to return to work. I

thought that I was looking fairly well, although several months afterward a few customers confessed that they were very concerned when I first started back because I looked so pale and had lost quite a bit of weight. While I was still in the hospital Dr. Abrams left the country for several months. While he was gone an incident happened with the doctor who was covering for him that still disturbs me. I had asked him when I could get back to my exercise program. He wanted to know what I had in mind and how much of it. I told him that I wanted to resume running, playing tennis, and swimming. He said that running was all right, to stay away from the tennis for a while longer, and not to swim. I asked why I couldn't play tennis and swim. He told me that tennis could disturb the healing process in the surgery site. He went on to tell me that, since there would probably be women and children in the pool, my appearance could upset them because of the very large and unsightly scar, which was still in the process of healing. I resented his reminder of my newly changed appearance and told him that I fully intended to wear a T-shirt when I swam. He said in that case it would be all right. Perhaps I was being too sensitive but his remark really hurt me. It was bad enough adjusting to having cancer without being told that my appearance was now offensive to others.

I started back on my exercise program. Getting into some physical activity and getting myself into a little better shape helped me physically but it was also probably the greatest thing I could have done for myself mentally.

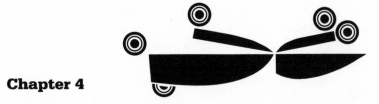

Chapter 4

My mother was in the process of moving into an apartment from the house that I grew up in and that she and my father had lived in for twenty-seven years. Going to New York under the guise of helping her pack and move, I thought that that

would be the best time for me to tell her what had happened.
On July 22, 1977, I flew into New York and she picked me up
at the airport. The timing of the move was perfect because I
felt I had to tell her what had transpired in person, not over
the phone. This seemed to be the ideal opportunity. She could
see for herself that I was fine and there really was nothing for
her to worry about. I must admit that it was a very, very difficult thing to do. How do you tell your mother that you have
cancer and that the outlook is not all that great? Surprisingly,
she took it very well, much better in fact than I had anticipated. She was upset that I hadn't told her sooner, so that she
could have helped out or just have been there in case we
needed her. I told her there really hadn't been any time. We
had to make the decision and act fast so that Dr. Abrams
could do the surgery. Under normal circumstances it might
have been nice to have had my mother there in order to help
Lynne, especially with Jared, and for both of them to just give
moral support to each other. However, the relationship between my wife and my mother wasn't that good to begin with
and I didn't feel there would be a great deal of moral support
given by either. Even though I love them both, I frankly didn't
feel that I needed the additional problem of having them together at a time when I couldn't be there as the mediator. The
day after I told Mom, her sister and her daughter, my aunt
and cousin, arrived from Louisville. They were on their way
to Connecticut and had stopped for a day for a visit. My
cousin Judy and I have always been very close and she has
been a tremendous boost to me through all this. Even though
she has had more than her share of personal problems, she
has always found time to be concerned and to lend moral
support. I think that their arriving when they did was a big
help to my mother because it gave her someone else to talk to
about the situation and maybe it cushioned the shock a little
for her.

Both Lynne and my mother decided to take the same attitude about the cancer. It was discovered, removed, and therefore gone forever. Because I had done my homework and researched the topic at the medical library at Michigan State

University, I was quite aware of how unrealistic this attitude was. I knew that the chances of a recurrence were very high and that I would have to go beyond five years without any sign of the cancer at all before my chances of survival would even begin to look reasonable. I didn't see any purpose in bursting the balloon that both Lynne and my mother had decided to ride on. I told them that I thought their attitude was fine but that I had decided to keep an open mind.

My knowledge of cancer has been developed through a gradual learning process. First there were the two forms of the basal cell and then the melanoma. When Dr. Wesley told me about the first basal cell I was more upset than I let anyone know at the time, if for no other reason than that just the word *cancer*, especially applied to me, scared the hell out of me. I researched the basal cell and learned that what Dr. Wesley had told me was true. If taken care of, it should be no more than a temporary minor nuisance. However, I did start to think about the actual ramifications of cancer and the tremendous impact that it can have on the person, his family, and those around him. I would eventually experience the full impact.

When Dr. Abrams told me about the melanoma and its consequences, I knew that this was no basal cell and that I really had a problem but I didn't realize how big it was. Fortunately, because of the urgency of scheduling the surgery so soon, I probably was more prepared than most people. Because of the experiences with the basal cells and the thinking I had done concerning cancer and its applications to me as an individual, I believe I was a little more mentally prepared to deal with the situation. In any case, because there was so little time from when the decision was made to the actual surgery, I really didn't have long to dwell on the subject or to get too worked up over it. I had a lot to get done in the two days before the operation and that kept me very busy. For most of the weekend Lynne had cried. I tried to console her and told her that everything would be fine, although, I wasn't at all sure myself.

After the operation, I started to learn more about what was in store for me. After leaving the hospital I read as much as I could find on melanoma at the medical library. I learned several things: that the chances of my living beyond five years were less than 20 percent; that the only predictable thing about malignant melanoma was its total unpredictability; and that there is very little known about it.

I wasn't about to throw in the towel but I did want to get my affairs in order just in case.

For the next several months things went along fairly well, no flare-ups, no problems. Dr. Abrams had been in contact with the National Cancer Research Institute again during this time and they advised getting an additional opinion after the surgery, even though they concurred with the treatment up to this point. They recommended that I go to one of the leading cancer centers on the East Coast. I was perfectly happy with things the way they were and saw no reason to take additional time off and spend nearly five hundred dollars—mostly travel expenses, which insurance does not cover but which are a medical deduction for tax purposes, plus what medical costs my insurance would not cover—just to get another opinion, especially since we already knew what they were going to say. However, Dr. Abrams said, "Look, Ken, do this for me. They just might have some sort of program that might be of some benefit to you. Even if they don't, do it so that I feel better about the whole situation and we have their opinion on record, OK?" What a mistake that turned out to be.

I arrived at the center at nine in the morning for a ten o'clock appointment as instructed. I saw three different secretaries, each asking to see the same insurance information, and was then passed on to the first nurse, who passed me on to another nurse, who passed me on to still another nurse, who finally said, "Sit over there," pointing to the waiting room, "until we call you." Two and a half hours later they called me. I went in to see the doctor and couldn't believe what happened next. After she introduced herself, the doctor asked what I was there for and what she could do for me. I was more than a little annoyed at this. Dr. Abrams had spent considerable time getting all my records and reports together and sent there; they contained all the pertinent data on what had transpired up to that point, on which these doctors were supposed to base their recommendations. Dr. Abrams had sent letters and made phone calls and had done all the preparatory work so that they would be familiar with my case and be prepared for me, and now this doctor asks what I was there for. I explained all this to the doctor and she said that she had not seen any of my records or any letters from Dr. Abrams. She said that she did concur that it was a malignant melanoma and that all the correct steps had been taken. This really made me angry. I had taken time off and had spent nearly five hundred dollars to go back East for a second opinion, just to be told that they concur without ever seeing my records or knowing anything at all about my case. Then she had the nerve to tell me that this wasn't even her specialty and if I would wait she would see if one of her colleagues, who specializes in the area of melanoma, would consent to see me. I waited for another hour and a half only to be told that, although the doctor was in, he couldn't see me until the next day and that I should report back at nine the following morning. I informed her that I didn't think I would be back to see her associate and I didn't think that the center had offered me anything but a lot of aggravation and I left. I just couldn't see wasting any more time and money. I flew back to East Lansing that night and vowed never to return to that place again. I went in to see Dr. Abrams the next day and he said that he didn't blame me for leaving, that he would have done the same thing. He was more than a little upset at the way I was treated, but he wanted to wait until he got a copy of her report before doing anything. He was even more upset when it was four months before a letter from the center came.

Chapter 5

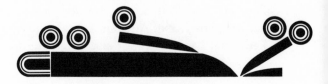

Things were going along great. I had completely recovered from the surgery and there had been no problem at all from a medical standpoint. I was working and doing well. In April of 1978, Lynne and I decided to take a little vacation during her spring break. The babysitter agreed to stay with Jared while we were gone. We flew down to Longboat Key on the west coast of Florida with some friends. A few days before we were to leave I had discovered a lump on the left side of my neck. I suspected that it was an enlarged lymph node and, given my history, was almost sure that it was another malignancy. I was also certain that another few days were not going to make a great deal of difference. We both, especially Lynne, needed a vacation. As I was learning, you don't ever get away from cancer; it is your silent partner in life, no matter where you go or what you do. Knowing this, I think I did fairly well, because nobody even suspected that there was anything wrong while we were on vacation. Lynne got a good rest and enjoyed the time away from the pressures she was under at home.

When we returned from Florida, I went in to see Dr. Abrams. He looked at the lump and scheduled a biopsy for later that week. There could not have been a more ominous sign at any time with the exception of the cancer spreading to a major organ. It would be proof that the cancer was still very much with me. I took this turn of events very well. Due to the research I had done, I always knew that the percentages were very high that there would be a recurrence at some time before the five-year period was up, most likely within the first eighteen months after the original surgery. I was concerned, however, with how Lynne and my mother would take the news. Their closed attitudes prevented any discussion of a recurrence because it was their position that the cancer was found, removed, and therefore gone forever. They were crushed when told of the possibility of the lump being malignant. I didn't want to take an I-told-you-so position but I did try to explain to them that the odds were always tremendously in favor of a recurrence and to think otherwise was great for them but foolhardy for me. I knew from my readings that, since the lymphatic system was one of the body's filtering systems, once the cancer hit that it would spread rapidly throughout the rest of my body. The only good news could be in the number of nodes that were affected. If fewer than five nodes were affected, there would be more reason to be optimistic than if more were involved. In either case the odds were now a lot less than they had been after the first surgery and then they were only 20 percent in my favor. Dr. Abrams told me that if this surgery was necessary it would be more serious and more complicated than the last one and that there would probably be some form of follow-up therapy. At the time, however, he was not sure what it would be or when it would get underway. The biopsy was performed and the results came in the following day. The surgery, a radical neck dissection, was scheduled for Wednesday, May 17. Before that all sorts of tests had to be performed in order to find out as much as was possible the full extent of the problem. Liver scan, bone scan, chest X ray, blood tests, and bone marrow tests were all done in the days leading up to the radical neck dissection. The surgery itself would involve an incision from under my chin around and up to my left ear and down to my left shoulder. All the lymph nodes, muscle, fat, tissue, and veins in the area would be removed. Things were to be removed that I didn't even know were there. After absorbing the initial shock of the lump being there and the biopsy, Lynne and my mother took the news that it was a malignancy fairly well. I called and informed my brother and he wanted to come down from Winnipeg, but I said no, that that was too much of an imposition and there really wasn't anything for him to do here. We did agree, though, to let my mother come this time. Jared was still only a little over two years old so there wasn't a lot that I could tell him. I did try to reassure him that I was just going to be away for a little while and that I would talk to him every day on the phone.

I entered the hospital on Tuesday, May 16, but this time they let me check in late in the afternoon to avoid any repeat of the first incident. The surgery was scheduled for the middle of the afternoon, so Lynne taught in the morning and came to the hospital right after lunch. Everyone was told what was going to happen and what to expect. I was probably going to be in intensive care for one or two days following the operation. Because of all the muscle that was going to be removed, I was told that I would probably lose a degree of mobility in my left arm. Dr. Abrams had consulted with the National Cancer Research Institute again and they concurred that this was the proper course of action.

Once more our friends were just great. They were there to help in any way they could. About an hour before I was to go down for the surgery I was given a shot to relax me. After they gave me the shot I was on the phone continuously, taking care of last-minute details for my business. When the surgical nurses arrived to take me down for the surgery, they had to wait for several minutes while I finished up with the Champion factory, checking on orders and making sure that certain things were done the way I wanted. I remember that, as I was rolling out of my room on the trip down to the operating room, four very close friends were there to stay with Lynne and my mother during the surgery. When I finally came out of intensive care over two days later, the same people were there again. It just happened that I came out of intensive care at about the same time that I went down for the surgery and their schedules permitted them to be with Lynne and my mother. I learned later that six other people had come by the night of the surgery at various times to stay with Lynne until midnight. My mother had had to leave earlier in the evening in order to stay with Jared after the babysitter left. After the surgery Dr. Abrams told Lynne that everything had gone well and that everyone should just keep their fingers crossed. It hadn't been necessary to do the tracheotomy that he had anticipated doing and that was good in that it was one less thing that my body had to deal with in the healing process. I only vaguely remember being awakened in the recovery room by the anesthesiologist and hearing his voice and several others in the background. From there I was taken directly to intensive care. I do remember waking up once there (I was kept sedated for the first two days) and seeing two nurses standing next to me and all the machinery with the blinking lights all around the area. The first solid memories that I have are of being taken out of intensive care and back to my room.

Several disturbing things happened while I was in the hospital this time. Three days after the surgery I started having a hard time breathing. I felt like I was slowly choking from an increasing pressure from within my neck at the surgery site. This continued for a few days but no one could figure out why. An eye, ear, nose, and throat specialist was called in but he could find no reason for the problem either. However, it was obvious that something was wrong. Finally, at about five one morning it became a real effort to breathe, my respirations were labored, and I had developed a fever. Dr. Abrams came to the hospital and inserted a tube down my throat to see if there was some sort of obstruction, but there wasn't. I mentioned to him that the surgery site had gotten as hard as a rock, that if he punched me there he would break his hand. After taking the bandages off and examining the wound, he knew at once what the problem was and why I was having trouble breathing. An internal infection had developed in the surgery site. It is very uncommon and Dr. Abrams said that he had seen it only a very few times in his career. He opened the site, drained it, and put me on antibiotics at once. I felt better within hours. The drugs brought my temperature down to normal and also started fighting the infection. It was explained that I really had been choking. No one could see what was happening because the infection was internal and the pressure was building inwardly.

During this stay in the hospital I became acquainted with an older man a few rooms down from mine. He also had cancer but he was obviously close to death. His family had come to visit him on a Sunday morning and then left for the rest of the day. He was taken down to the X-ray lab late in the morning. Whoever took him there must have just wheeled him down and left without checking with anyone. A few hours later one of the nurses commented that he had been down there a long time. I guess everyone just assumed that they weren't done with him yet. Another hour went by and one of the nurses said that she would check on him on her way down for her break. When she got there she found him still lying on the stretcher right where he had been left. The X-ray lab was closed and no one even knew that he was there. He was brought back to his room, where he died a few hours later. This really bothered me. I thought that was a really rotten way to spend your last hours, alone on a stretcher in a hospital hallway. I saw his family that evening but never said anything about it. I'm not sure what the point would have been in telling them. It would have only made them feel worse. I learned later that the person who had left him there lost her job. In defense of the nurses, I think that if they hadn't been so overworked at the time maybe someone would have realized sooner that something was wrong. Overall, I must say that the nursing care I have received in the hospital has been exceptional each and every time I have been there.

On the night of the sixteenth, the night before the surgery, I had called home to see how everything was going. I knew that Jared hadn't been feeling very well that day and I wanted to make sure that he was reassured about what was going on with me as I didn't know when I would be able to speak with him again. I called several times but no one answered and after about an hour I started to get concerned. I knew that if Jared wasn't feeling well and Lynne had to get him to a doctor she would probably come to the emergency room at the hospital I was in. I decided to just take a chance and went down to the emergency room, and, sure enough, Jared, Lynne, and my mother were all sitting there. They had not seen the doctor yet, so I sat down in my hospital gown and waited with them. I think that this made Jared feel a little more secure too. While we were sitting there waiting to see the doctor I started to hear over the paging system, "Would Mr. Kenneth Shapiro please report back to his room at once." Since I thought it was more important to stay with Jared at that time, I just ignored the calls. After seeing the doctor and finding out that Jared had a bad case of tonsillitis but would be just fine after he started taking some medication that the doctor prescribed, I got into a fight with my mother. Lynne had told her I planned on having a vasectomy at the same time as the radical neck surgery and she was vehemently against it. I told her that I wasn't going to stand there in a hospital gown in the emergency room while half the hospital was searching for me and fight with her about it, and I went back to my room after kissing Jared good-night. To say the staff was mad as hell would be an understatement. Several technicians were just standing around who were supposed to be giving me certain preoperative tests and getting me prepped for surgery while everyone else was out looking for me.

Lynne and I had discussed the implications of this recurrence of the cancer and what impact it was going to have on us. I had put forth the idea that I didn't think we should have any more children under these circumstances. It wouldn't be fair to anyone involved, especially another child, who might come into the world and have its father die within the first few years of its life. We discussed this and decided that it would probably be best if I had a vasectomy. Not that we were sure I was going to die because of this recurrence but the five-year prognosis, which wasn't great to begin with, was worse now. Even if I didn't die, by the time it would be safe for me to have another child I would probably be in my mid-forties. All things considered, I think that the right decision was made. I spoke with Dr. Abrams about it and asked him if it was possible to get this done at the same time as the radical neck dissection. I figured why not do it then since I was going to be under a general anesthetic—why not get both things out of the way at the same time. Also, if you're going to feel lousy from surgery anyway, why not feel lousy once and get it all out of the way rather than feeling lousy twice. He said it was rather unusual but he didn't see why it couldn't be done. He set it up with the surgeon who would do the vasectomy and they coordinated all the details.

I had hoped that my mother's being at the house and helping with Jared would make things a little easier for Lynne, but I was wrong. I wasn't back in my room for a full day when I started getting phone calls, first from Lynne and then from

my mother, each telling me what the other was doing wrong.
This bickering went on for several days, especially when they came to visit. I couldn't believe what was happening. I was lying in a hospital bed trying to recoup from surgery and my wife and my mother were arguing about petty, minor, stupid things. Early one morning Dr. Johnson came into my room, pulled up a chair, and said, "Ken, the last thing in the world that you need right now is problems with your family. Normally I wouldn't say anything, but because I am so close to you and your family, I can see that it is affecting you and therefore your recovery. Since I know that it is also affecting Lynne, Jared, and your mother, I think that something must be done, but for the life of me I don't know what." I said that I knew and that I would take care of it that day. I called my mother and asked her to come over to the hospital. When she arrived I asked her to return to New York. I thanked her very much for coming; however, I just couldn't let the situation between her and Lynne go on any longer. It wasn't working out for anyone, especially me. I should have realized this in the first place given the history of their relationship and the added strain of the surgery and cancer. I know that neither one of them meant any harm and that they both thought they were doing the right thing.

Before I left the hospital Dr. Abrams told me that he had discussed my situation with Dr. Johnson, Dr. Wesley (in an area the size of Lansing/East Lansing the private physicians comprise the hospital staff; they are one and the same), Dr. Norom, a local oncologist, and the NCRI. Everyone agreed there should be some form of follow-up therapy in order to try to inhibit any further spread of the cancer. However, no one was certain what the correct approach should be. Dr. Norom had recommended one course of action but the NCRI had recommended something else. The NCRI also recommended that I go to M. D. Anderson Hospital and Tumor Institute in Houston, Texas, for further consultation and possible therapy. Dr. Abrams said that he had taken the liberty of starting the process of getting me an appointment there as soon as possible. He tried to head off my objections by saying that he would do everything possible to avoid another fiasco such as the one I had at the East Coast center. I was firmly against this course of action but Dr. Abrams, Dr. Johnson, and Dr. Wesley were all firmly in favor of it.

Thus, on Sunday, June 11, 1978, I left for Houston for the first time. Lynne and I had decided that it would be best if she stayed with Jared so that both of us weren't gone.

Chapter 6

While I was at the airport in Lansing waiting to board the plane for Chicago, a friend came over and said that he was on this flight too. He had called me several times while I was in the hospital but this was the first time I had seen him since I had gotten out. He asked me how I was feeling and for the one and only time during this whole cancer business I said, "Lousy." I really don't know why I said it. It was true but it was very unlike me to say something like that to anyone other than one of my doctors. I think I made myself feel even worse by saying that. We had a nice visit on the flight from Lansing to Chicago and there we split up. I was flying on Delta and I had to change terminals, which meant I also had to go through the X-ray machines again. I was carrying about a dozen X rays and a box of medical slides from the biopsies and operations of the past eighteen months. In Lansing I explained what these were and asked if they would visually examine them rather than put them through the machines. They very courteously agreed and there were no problems. In Chicago they wouldn't even consider it. I asked to speak with the supervisor and they wouldn't let me do that either. I was told that if I wanted to get on a plane the hand-carried items would have to go through the machines no matter what they were. I was afraid the machines would alter or have some effect on the X rays and slides. I was furious but I didn't seem to have too much choice in the matter, so after a lot of arguing I had to give in.

I landed in Houston at about ten in the evening and the temperature was still about eighty-five degrees and the humidity was even higher. Since this was my first trip to Houston, I didn't know a thing about the city, where anything was or how to get there. When I had made my hotel reservations I asked the woman on the phone and she told me that there were buses that ran from Intercontinental Airport right to the hotel where I was going to be staying. I asked around and found out where I could get that bus. The ride took about an hour with other stops along the way. The last stop was the Shamrock Hilton Hotel, where I was going to stay for the first night. It was about twelve-thirty in the morning when we finally arrived and all the restaurants and snack bars were closed as was room service in the hotel. I found a vending machine, got a candy bar and a Coke, and then went to sleep.

I stayed at the Shamrock that first night, but in the morning I switched over to the Anderson Mayfair as had been prearranged. After registering there I started my check-in process for the hospital. They were not only expecting me and waiting for me, they were ready and willing to answer my questions fully and honestly. I was shown a short orientation film that explained what M. D. Anderson Hospital is and what they try to accomplish there. The film explained that M.D.A. is a big place, that the outpatient clinic alone sees over twelve hundred people each and every day. As much as they try to avoid it, waiting is usually necessary in order to take each person individually and do the best possible job. I appreciated this. They tell you what to expect, that they will do their best to be on time, but that it is more important to be thorough than it is to be fast. After the film I had a complete examination from head to toe. From there I was sent across the street to the main part of the hospital, where I was to meet a guide. This was not special attention. They have a staff of people whose sole job it is to direct or assist new patients or other patients who have a hard time getting around. I reported to the information desk and told the receptionist that I was to have "Doris" paged. They called her and I figured that I would be waiting for awhile, so I settled down with some paperwork that I had brought along. I had just gotten my briefcase opened and taken some papers out when Doris walked up. She introduced herself and explained what we were going to be doing. We started the trip at the patient routing desk and from there went to the different stations for the blood tests, liver scan, brain scan, chest X rays, and so on. It took about two hours and by three o'clock I was done for the day. I was amazed at the efficiency of this huge place and how the staff was totally prepared at each station. There was a minimum of waiting. The longest I had to wait was at the scanning stations and this was owing to the time required for the injected radioactive substance to reach the part of the body to be scanned. Other than that there was never more than a five-to-ten-minute wait for any test. After we were done Doris told me where to meet her the following morning. She made me feel much more comfortable and at ease in this new situation. M.D.A. is such a large place that its sheer size alone can intimidate you.

Since I was done for the day I went down to the cafeteria and got a snack. From there I decided to look around the place and see for myself what was where and to just orientate myself to these surroundings. Actually, Anderson is in a complex of hospitals called the Texas Medical Center. It has got to be a doctor's delight. It is a smorgasbord of almost everything in medicine. After that I went back to the Mayfair and just relaxed and took it easy for awhile. I called Lynne and Jared and told them everything that had happened that day. Both Lynne and I were relieved that this was going to be much different from my previous experience with a major medical center. That evening I had dinner in my room, went to bed very early, and got a good night's sleep. I needed it.

The next day Doris took me to see Dr. Fredericks, who was going to be in charge of my case. I had to wait, but because I had been forewarned and knew why it was happening, the wait didn't bother me. When he finally arrived, Dr. Fredericks had all my test results from the previous day, all the records I had brought down there with me, M.D.A.'s own analysis of the X rays and slides I had brought with me, and all the information that Dr. Abrams had sent. He examined me, went over all the results of the tests I had taken, and asked many questions. I don't think that he was prepared for me, though. I have this habit of insisting on knowing everything and insisting on answers to questions that sometimes really can't be answered, such as, what's going to happen next, and when? How long do I have to live? Do I have any chance at all of beating it? Dr. Fredericks said very calmly, "Mr. Shapiro, you seem to attribute powers to me that I do not possess. Most of the questions you have asked me have no ready answers. I can give you my opinion, but that is all it is, my opinion, for whatever that's worth." I replied that his best opinion was exactly what I wanted. He told me that if I could pass the five-year period, he would be very optimistic about my chances of survival, although, quite candidly, the chances of my getting through a five-year period without any recurrences were very slim. Therefore, he would do the best he could in treating the cancer and keeping it in check as well as he could for as long as possible.

It is M.D.A.'s philosophy to treat cancer very aggressively, whenever possible. Because I was strong and in relatively good condition, I was considered a good candidate. Dr. Fredericks explained to me that not much was known about malignant melanoma in the higher stages or how to treat it. He went on to tell me that their treatment of choice was an experimental program that would be very unpleasant at best. The side effects are bad, and as the results were coming in it seemed that those who had the worst side effects were the ones who seemed to be responding the best. Therefore, it seemed that the worse the side effects were the better it was. He said the results they were getting were encouraging but certainly not spectacular. He explained he did not think that this was going to be the final cure for melanoma but that it was going to be one more step in the right direction.

It is important to understand why I agreed to this method of treatment in the first place. You don't go to a place like M. D. Anderson just to refuse their best treatment. You have to go with their best judgment. Because of my strength, mental toughness, and stubborn streak, I figured that if other people had gone through this I should be able to get through it too without too many problems. I have always felt that I could withstand physical discomfort (i.e., pain) better than most people and that I could withstand it this time. These personality traits were nothing new. As a child, I was always the one to take up the dare that someone offered, and I was usually successful at it. In athletics I would work twice as hard as others and often excelled over people who were bigger, stronger, and more talented than I. I am the same way in business. I always tackle the big customers, go for the big orders, and stand my ground against the competition. But there are things in life that, no matter how strong you are and how tough you are, you aren't going to beat.

Dr. Fredericks explained the treatment plan, answered my questions, and then took me over to the immunotherapy station and introduced me to Madeline, the nurse in charge of implementing this program with the patients. She went over the entire written part of the program with me and explained anything that I didn't understand. She told me the drugs were very closely regulated by the government and could only be obtained from one of the three research facilities that were experimenting with them at the time. She gave me a supply of the drugs with all the written instructions regarding dosage and their administration. I was to take them back home with me and report to Dr. Norom. Madeline told me not to hesitate to call her or Dr. Fredericks if I had any questions or problems regarding the treatments. She also provided me with some forms. Each day that I took a treatment I was to keep track of the side effects on an almost hourly basis. If compiled and published, they would make a horror story that few, if any, would believe.

The treatment program called for a combination of immunotherapy and chemotherapy. The drugs used are:

Immunotherapy—C-Parvum
Chemotherapy—DTIC and Actinomycin D

They should be given as follows: C-Parvum is given intra-
venously in 150cc normal saline through a special filter over at
least one hour daily for fourteen days as follows:

0.55 mgm on days 1 and 2
1.1 mgm on day 3
2.2 mgm on day 4
4.4 mgm on days 5 through 14

Chemotherapy should then be given on days 15 through 19
as follows: Actinomycin D 3.3 mgm in 50cc D5WIV (solution
of 5% dextrose and water) over fifteen to twenty minutes, followed by DTIC 500 mgm in 100cc D5WIV over thirty to forty-
five minutes.

C-Parvum should then be given in 4.4 mgm (divided into
several sites, such as left arm, right arm, left leg, right leg,
etc.) on days 7, 12, and 17 of each twenty-two–day course of
chemotherapy. At the completion of three twenty-two–day
courses of chemotherapy, another fourteen-day course of C-
Parvum is given.

I left knowing what the program consisted of and that the
side effects would be unpleasant but should not last any longer
than six hours. I was apprehensive, to be sure, though confident that my strength and mental toughness would help me
through it.

After two days in Houston I checked out of the Mayfair and
headed back to East Lansing. My main thoughts were on my
cancer, M. D. Anderson Hospital, the medication that I was
carrying and how I was going to get through the X-ray machines, my family, and my work, in particular something that
I said to Dr. Fredericks regarding my job. I told him that if I
could work during the treatment I could get through it but
that if it turned out that I couldn't work then I would have to
stop the treatment. This worried me.

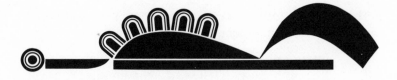

Chapter 7

Drs. Abrams and Johnson thought that Dr. Norom would be the best one to handle this part of my treatment. He was a local oncologist who had an excellent reputation and was highly recommended by his contemporaries. Since I didn't know a thing about him I really had no choice, I thought, but to take the recommendation of my doctors. It would be my first encounter with medical jealousies and the most hideous form of discrimination that I can think of, medical politics. Before I left Houston, Dr. Fredericks warned me not to be surprised if Dr. Norom wasn't too enthusiastic about this program. Because he was at a facility that was also conducting cancer research, he might not like working on programs and protocols from another research facility. It never really dawned on me that would or could occur. After all, these are professionals—physicians—their primary concern should be the patient's well-being. Sure enough, Dr. Norom made no bones about the fact that he didn't like the program, knew nothing about the drug or how to administer it, and it was only because Dr. Abrams and Dr. Johnson prevailed upon him that he agreed to take this on. He said he was against my going to Houston in the first place, that they didn't have any more answers than anybody else. However, I wondered, if he didn't know anything about the program or the drug how could he be so critical of it?

While I was in Texas, Lynne had met the mother of a child in Jared's nursery school class. In the course of the conversation Lynne mentioned where I was and why. She learned that this woman's husband was an oncologist and was very familiar with M.D.A. and many of the doctors there. Lynne urged me to call her husband, Dr. Kenyon, but I was hesitant about

getting another physician involved. However, I did ask Dr.
Norom and one of his associates if they knew Dr. Kenyon and
both went into a tirade that made him sound just a little to the
left of Jack the Ripper. I assumed that he must really be a bad
doctor if his contemporaries thought so poorly of him. I had
never heard a doctor criticize another doctor as severely and
completely as they did. I have learned through experience
that, in general, when there is such intense dislike and criti-
cism as that shown by Dr. Norom and his associate it is usually more personal than professional and factual.

My game plan was to take the treatments each day at three
in the afternoon, go directly home, work for an hour, go
through the side effects for six or seven hours, recover, get
some sleep, and be ready to work the next morning. It was
important to me—more than important, it was vital—to be
able to work through this whole thing, as I had explained to
Dr. Fredericks before agreeing to the experimental program.
He told me that it would be difficult at times but he thought it
could be done if I was that determined.

On Thursday, June 22, 1978, at 2:00 P.M., I reported to the
clinic where Dr. Norom was for my first treatment. I had to
report early this time because there was an hour's worth of
tests that had to be done before the first treatment. When I
arrived I was surprised to learn that Dr. Norom was not there
but that he would try to get back before the treatment was
over. The head nurse arrived and assured me that she had
read over the protocols several times and that she was sure
she could handle it. She then proceeded to ask me questions
about the protocols and the instructions that I had received in
Houston. Rather nervously I permitted her to administer the
C-Parvum. After the treatment I waited for a while, hoping
that Dr. Norom would return. He never did. I went home still
unsure that I had been given the C-Parvum correctly or what
was about to happen, although I felt confident I could handle
anything. Around 4:30, about an hour and a half after the
treatment had ended, I started to feel achy, as if I were coming down with the flu, and went upstairs to lie down. This

44 was the beginning of what was to be one of the worst nights and days of my life. I would also learn that not all members of the medical profession are the all-knowing, all-caring, compassionate group that people think they are. I feel very fortunate to have the team of doctors that I now have; they are all first-class, top-notch professionals. Dr. Norom was another story.

After the flulike feeling, the side effects started getting worse. The achiness persisted and the chills began. They started slowly and built up. I got under the covers, used a heating pad, and put on two sweat suits, sweat socks, jackets; nothing helped. I got into the shower and slowly turned the cold water off until I had nothing but the hot water running and I was still shivering. Nothing seemed to help. My teeth were chattering so fast and so hard that we couldn't even get a temperature reading for fear the thermometer would snap. After two hours, the chills broke and I started getting warmer and warmer until my temperature hit 104 degrees. We applied ice packs. I got back into the shower and used only the cold water to try to cool off and bring the temperature down. Aspirin was strictly forbidden with this type of therapy and Tylenol didn't help at all. Another two hours passed and the fever broke. I started feeling better and thought that it was over for this first night. I knew that the side effects I had experienced were stronger than normally expected and I had been told that the worse the side effects the better it is. Since the drugs must then be working, I was actually encouraged. I thought that I had made it through this first session quite well. Since we didn't know what to expect this first night, Lynne had asked a friend to stay over in order to help out with Jared in case Lynne had problems with me. As far as I know he never knew about anything that was going on. Lynne was with me and Jared played until it was time for him to go to sleep for the night.

Half an hour later everything started happening again, n more severely this time. The achiness felt as if my joints swollen to three times their normal size. The chills hit and no matter what I did I couldn't get warm. I was shaking so badly that I was almost levitating off the bed. They lasted an hour and again I went directly into a fever running in the 102°–103° range. This also lasted about an hour and then broke. By this time we began to worry. Lynne tried calling Dr. Norom, only to find out that his clinic does not have night hours but that if we wanted to leave a message the operator would try to reach him at home. An hour later Dr. Norom returned our call and after hearing about the problems I was having said to take a couple of Tylenol and get some sleep. I took four more Tylenol and after a short time the whole process started again. It was exactly like the previous two. I knew something was wrong. The side effects were supposed to be bad but once they were over they were supposed to be over for good. Lynne called Dr. Norom again, by calling the operator at the clinic and leaving a message, and at six in the morning he returned our call. Lynne told him that we couldn't get the side effects to stop. He suggested that I take a tranquilizer and get some sleep. I began to feel that he didn't know what to do and that I was more or less on my own. That cycle ended only to have another one start half an hour later. Lynne got angry and called Dr. Norom again, saying that something had to be done. This time Dr. Norom unloaded on her, saying that he was against this from the very start, he thought we were wrong in going to Houston, he'd never even heard of this drug before, and he had no idea of what to do. We really *were* on our own.

I decided to try to wait it out, call Houston, and see what they wanted to do. When it hit again I noticed that it wasn't as severe or as long lasting. I even managed to fall asleep for an hour before being awakened by another round of the chills and fever. Lynne tried calling Dr. Kenyon, this time without telling me. She had already taken the day off from work and the babysitter had arrived to take care of Jared. Dr. Kenyon returned her call about ten minutes later from the hospital. Lynne explained who we were and what was happening. I then got on the phone and described the side effects. Dr. Kenyon, who was familiar with C-Parvum, said something was severely wrong. He sent one of his P.A.'s (physician's assistant) over to our house. The P.A. gave me an I.V. of something that seemed to help a little. He wanted me to go directly to the hospital, but I wanted to see Dr. Abrams first. Lynne drove me over to Dr. Abrams' office and, since he was on his way from the hospital, his nurse put us right into one of the examining rooms that had a couch in it so I could lie down as I was still quite unsteady.

When Dr. Abrams walked in he took one look at me and said, "O my God, what happened to you?" We explained everything to him and he wanted to hospitalize me immediately. We explained what Dr. Kenyon wanted to do and he called Dr. Kenyon. After conferring, both of them agreed that if Dr. Kenyon couldn't pull me out of this cycle I was in by five that afternoon I would be hospitalized until they could come up with the answer. Dr. Kenyon told me that another C-Parvum treatment right now could be fatal and I should wait at least two weeks to give my body a chance to recover from its current ordeal. The C-Parvum finally worked itself out of my system with the aid of the drugs that Dr. Kenyon kept giving me I.V. By late afternoon I was showing enough improvement that both Dr. Abrams and Dr. Kenyon agreed to let me go home. To this day no one knows for sure what happened in that first treatment. The prevailing opinion is that I was given approximately ten times the prescribed dosage I should have received and my body reacted violently. There is no excuse for what happened, although this type of mistake easily occurs if the person handling the drug is not familiar with the way it is packaged. Apparently, C-Parvum is packaged in such a way that it has to be divided by ten in order to get the proper dosage. If the person handling it is not familiar with this and isn't paying attention to details, an overdose is the result—as happened with me.

I still shudder every time I think about that episode. I learned some valuable lessons, such as making sure the people know what they are doing regardless of the prestige of the hospital or the reputation of the staff. You must make sure that you fully understand what is going to happen and what the normal boundaries of the side effects are, and what to do in the event these boundaries are crossed and something goes **47** wrong. Avoid medical clinics that operate on a nine-to-five basis. They are certainly not the place for the treatment of cancer, or anything else that possibly might need twenty-four–hour control. You must always be able to contact the physician in charge no matter what time it is or what day it is. The feeling of not being able to contact the physician in charge or anyone at all who might be able to help during an incident such as this is one of sheer terror, not knowing what is going to happen next or what to do about it. It's a feeling that I hope to never experience again or that anyone should have to experience. Obviously, I got rid of Dr. Norom immediately.

My decision to switch to Dr. Kenyon was not very popular with my other doctors. Dr. Kenyon was considered a nonconformist to the local medical politics and the etiquettes of medicine. All I cared about, however, was good treatment and Dr. Kenyon has more than justified my confidence in him. I learned firsthand that medical politics are cruel and vicious. The fact that a few people will die here and there because one hospital administrator or one doctor is upset with another doctor seems to make no difference whatsoever. An example of this occurred when I switched to Dr. Kenyon. I wanted to use the hospital that Dr. Abrams was affiliated with so he could help monitor my treatment. Approval had to be given in order for the C-Parvum to be used in that hospital. It was taken before the medical board but they would not authorize its use as presented because it was an experimental drug. However, they informed me that if I would permit one of their top staff oncologists to administer the drug they would approve its use. When I inquired into who it was they had in mind, they told me Dr. Norom would be the one. In other words, Dr. Norom had more political clout than Dr. Kenyon. He managed to bar the use of C-Parvum by Dr. Kenyon in the hospital of my choice. I went with Dr. Kenyon to his small hospital. I wasn't pleased about it at all. As a matter of fact, I was very nervous about it. However, as long as he was around the treatment was very good. When he wasn't around the treatment wasn't as good. He had given me his home phone number, though, to use when he wasn't present in the hospital. All my local doctors refused to work with Dr. Kenyon except for one, Dr. Abrams of course. He is always there for me regardless of the political aspects of the situation.

I waited the two weeks recommended by Dr. Kenyon before starting my treatments again. During that time he informed Houston that he had taken over the administration of my treatments. Also during this time Lynne and I fully discussed this first episode and we decided that, if there were not better controls on the administration of the C-Parvum plus assurances that qualified medical personnel would be available in case of problems, this program was not going to be for us. I would be far better off on my own than to have to go through more uncontrolled, unsupervised treatments. There would also be no way in the world for me to be able to work during treatments that had side effects as severe as those I had just experienced. I again stated that if I could work through it I could get through it, but that if I couldn't work I would have to get off the program.

During that two-week period Dr. Lewis, one of Dr. Kenyon's associate physicians, checked with the UCLA medical school. She knew that they had been doing some work with C-Parvum. They told her of an interesting experiment they had done concerning the use of steroids to block the side effects of the C-Parvum while not blocking the effectiveness of the drug itself. Dr. Kenyon and Dr. Lewis developed a program for me along the lines of the UCLA program. It required using a certain amount of the steroid and halving it each day as the C-Parvum was doubled for the first five days and then discontinuing the use of the steroid altogether. It made sense to block the side effects if possible while not diminishing the effectiveness of the C-Parvum. After all, I am not a glutton for punishment.

Dr. Kenyon had another patient who had malignant melanoma who went to M.D.A. for her surgery and follow-up treatment. She, too, was on the C-Parvum treatment. As far as we could tell, we were the only two people in the Midwest on this drug. I spoke with her at great length on the phone

one evening. She said she'd had no problems with the C-
Parvum. She would take the treatment, return home, go to
bed for a few hours, get very mild side effects during that
time, and then get up and go out for the evening. She couldn't
believe my first experience with the C-Parvum and said that I
must have gotten the overdose that everyone had suspected.
After our discussion I felt confident that it would be much
easier from that point on. Plus I felt greatly relieved that Dr.
Kenyon did indeed know how to administer C-Parvum and
that either he or Dr. Lewis was always either on duty or in
contact with the hospital in case of problems. Dr. Kenyon and
I discussed the differences between her reactions to the C-
Parvum and mine and he warned me that just because she
didn't get serious side effects from the drug was no guarantee
that I wouldn't. The drug reacts differently on different people
and individual responses could not be predicted. He recommended that I be hospitalized for the first five days of the
treatment so the side effects could be closely monitored. I
agreed wholeheartedly. I wanted to avoid at all costs another
episode like the first one.

I planned to check into the hospital where Dr. Kenyon
was late on a Wednesday and get the first treatment that evening. That way I could minimize my loss of work time and
utilize the weekends as treatment days. Dr. Kenyon arranged
all this for me and in general just tried to make things easier,
for which I am very grateful. In contrast, Dr. Norom never
considered my wishes. He even had the outright gall to say
that on weekends or when any holiday came about I would
have to get enough of the drug the day before, so that I could
keep it refrigerated and then take it to one of the hospital
emergency rooms and have the treatment administered by
someone who was on duty at the time. His clinic was closed
after five during the week and not opened at all on weekends
or holidays. At the time, I didn't know any better and was
going to do exactly as I was told. Looking back at that now, it
still scares the hell out of me just thinking about walking into
an emergency room with this drug that no one knows anything about or even heard of and saying, "Hi, here I am. How

would you like to give me a treatment with this experimental drug?" It's absolutely incredible he would even suggest such a thing, but he obviously wanted his evenings, weekends, and holidays free. Maybe certain types of medicine can be practiced this way, but I guarantee you that cancer treatment is not one of them. Especially when the daily use of drugs is involved.

I want to strongly emphasize that the problems I ran into could have been avoided had I questioned Dr. Norom the way I would question any physician I work with now. However, that was my first experience with something like that and I didn't know any better. I was going on the advice of my doctors, who honestly thought Dr. Norom could handle the situation. My major complaint with Dr. Norom is not that there was a mistake apparently made in the administration of the drug, but that he didn't even think it was important enough for him to be present to oversee the administering of this drug that even he was unfamiliar with and let someone else, who knew less than he, do it. When problems started occurring he didn't even attempt to do anything to help and virtually abandoned me at the height of problems that could have been life threatening. My advice to all who might find themselves in a similar situation is, first of all, learn as much as possible about the physician administering the treatment and what he or she knows, if anything, about it and, second, make sure they are at a facility that is open and staffed twenty-four hours a day with people who can handle any problem that occurs.

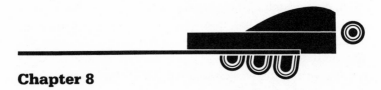

Chapter 8

I checked into the hospital late Wednesday afternoon, July 19. After the standard blood tests, blood pressure measurement, and so on, an I.V. infusion of normal saline solution was established. The steroid was administered first and the C-Parvum

immediately afterward. Everything went just beautifully.
After both drugs were given, the I.V. was left in place so that
an open vein was immediately available in case of severe side
effects. What I was unaware of at the time was that there was
no antidote that would work on me. Lynne and I had discussed the situation and even though we were both still a
little nervous about starting the treatments again and being in
this hospital, which was known more for abortions that had
been performed there than for cancer treatment, we decided
that it would be best for her to stay home with Jared. He was
still only two and a half years old and his need for his mother
at the time, we felt, was more important than mine. However,
a good friend did come and stay with me well into the night to
make sure that everything was going well and that there was
proper supervision and care. He was reporting back to Lynne
and easing her fears, also.

The first treatment was a breeze. All I experienced was
a slight elevation in temperature. The next four treatments
were also easy. As the C-Parvum was doubled and the steroid
halved each day, there was a slight increase in the side effects
though never to the point I couldn't handle them with ease,
and once they were over they were over for the rest the day. I
felt that this was more like it and more the way I had anticipated it being. I was released on Sunday after my treatment
and would return each day at three for another treatment.
Monday, the sixth treatment was the first without the steroid
and I returned home feeling confident that I could handle
what lay ahead.

After I arrived home I did some work for a little while, then
played with Jared until I started to feel a little achy and went
upstairs to lie down. Dr. Kenyon and Dr. Lewis both had told
me that the side effects would probably be slightly worse this
night since we had eliminated the steroid completely. They
explained that my body had had enough time to adjust to the
C-Parvum during the previous five days and should now be
accustomed to its presence. I would probably experience only
slightly worsened side effects. The achiness continued and
the chills arrived. They steadily worsened until I was again

almost levitating off the bed. I was determined to fight it. The chills lasted about ninety minutes and turned immediately into fever. We were monitoring and recording my temperature every half-hour. My temperature hit 103 degrees and remained there for an hour and then broke. After that I started feeling better, exhausted, but better. I was nervous though; this was more than just slightly worse than the previous five days. I wasn't sure if it really was over for the night or if it was going to return as it had in my first experience with the C-Parvum. There was no recurrence and I got a few hours' sleep and went to work in the morning.

I reported in at three the next afternoon for my treatment and related the previous night's experience to Dr. Kenyon. He wasn't pleased and wanted to be notified if the reactions got that bad again. I took the next treatment and the chills and fever were worse than the previous night. The side effects lasted about four hours with the chills worse than the night before and the fever hitting 104 degrees. We had some difficulty locating Dr. Kenyon as he was not at home or at the hospital and when he called back the side effects had subsided. I wanted him to call Houston first thing in the morning to see if these side effects were within reason and how they wanted us to proceed. He agreed. I went to work in the morning and reported in at three to see what Houston had said and what we were going to do. Dr. Fredericks said that we had not followed the protocols and he did not agree with the UCLA study using steroids to block the side effects. The steroids act as immunodepressants and the purpose of the C-Parvum is to act as an immunostimulant. He didn't feel it was wise or logical to use steroids, and since the drug was under their control it was to be used as they had prescribed or they would "pull the treatment." Dr. Fredericks said that the only known antidote that was permissible to be used for the C-Parvum was morphine. I wasn't happy about this because the first thing that I had thought of was to go back to the use of the steroid in order to block the side effects. However, I must admit that what Dr. Fredericks said did make sense. Why depress the very system that you are trying to stimulate?

Throughout my research, the preponderance of the published material seemed to be coming from M. D. Anderson Hospital and I had become a believer in immunotherapy. To this day I believe that somewhere within the human immunological system is the answer to every disease in the world and that if we only understood how our immunological system worked we would know that in order to cure such and such disease we must plug such and such into the body to alert the immunologic system to wake up and send out the necessary killer cells to combat the disease-causing cells. However, since the science of immunology is so young, we really don't understand that much about it. Much research is still needed to understand why the system does what it does and, possibly even more important, why it doesn't do what it is supposed to do at certain times.

Morphine, though, is another story. Dr. Kenyon and I discussed the likelihood of my becoming addicted to the narcotic. He told me that the odds of addiction were very high because the dosage needed to combat the side effects of the C-Parvum was very high. My choices were taking the C-Parvum without the morphine and risking the side effects, which were getting worse and could themselves be harmful, or using morphine and risk becoming an addict. It was not as cut and dried a decision as that though. I considered what would happen if I did become an addict. How could I work? How could I function? How could I face anyone knowing that I was an addict no matter what the reason was? On the other hand, how could I not give it a chance? It didn't make any sense to try to "tough it out" only to die from complications from the treatment, such as a heart attack. If morphine was the only way this treatment could be given the chance to work, then that would have to be the way to go. I decided to try the C-Parvum straight one more time, but, if the side effects were still as bad or got worse, I would try the morphine and take the risk of narcotic addiction.

I took the eighth treatment without the morphine or the steroid and returned home to await another night of chills and fever. This was worse than any of the previous nights.

My temperature hit 105.3 degrees. I had always been under the impression that at that temperature level there would be brain damage, but I discovered later that as long as ice packs were used continuously there was little danger. Constant monitoring was necessary though. I can attest that a 105-degree temperature does get a little uncomfortable. Sleep finally came and I went to work in the morning. After discussing it with Dr. Kenyon I decided to try the morphine. It was getting increasingly difficult to put up with the chills and fever and the exhaustion that followed every night. I knew I couldn't keep going this way and I was feeling that I was in more danger continuing in this manner with the drug than I was with the cancer itself. I called Lynne and told her about the decision. She had to pick me up at the hospital since I was not going to be in any condition to drive. Once the decision had been made and there was nothing I could do about the results, I decided that I might just as well try to enjoy it. I could find out firsthand what it felt like to be totally "spaced out." I was given the C-Parvum; we waited about forty-five minutes before the achiness started. Dr. Kenyon gave me a large dose of morphine and within fifteen minutes I was feeling very lightheaded. I sort of floated out of the hospital under the guidance of Lynne and some of the hospital staff. I don't remember much of that evening except vomiting a few times. I went to work in the morning not knowing what to expect. Dr. Kenyon thought that the vomiting was caused by something other than the morphine. If I had taken the morphine on an empty stomach it could produce the same reaction. Whatever the reason, since it had blocked the chills and fever, and the vomiting was not severe, I decided to keep taking the morphine.

I received my next dose of C-Parvum that day and as soon as the achiness began I was again pumped full of morphine. We waited ten minutes and when I got up to leave I was still in full control of all my faculties, both mental and physical. Dr. Kenyon thought it would just take a little longer to work and encouraged me to go home, climb in bed, and get some sleep. I went home, climbed into bed, but never went to sleep.

The morphine never clicked. I was aware of everything going on around me, no high or spaced-out feeling, and, worst of all, it was ineffective in blocking the side effects. The achy feeling got worse and the chills hit with such ferocity that I could not control my limbs and was shaking the whole bed. Lynne called the hospital but Dr. Kenyon had already left. She left messages at both the hospital and his home to call at once. Half an hour later I told Lynne to call the hospital again and tell them that I was coming in. They suggested sending an ambulance or the police to come and get me, but I chattered that I didn't want to wait any longer and I would make it down there by myself. Remember, I am stronger and tougher than everyone else, also sometimes dumber. Lynne wanted to drive me but there was no one around who could stay with Jared and I still did not want him seeing me in this condition. It was 96 degrees outside and I stumbled to the car dressed in a heavy-weight hooded sweatshirt, sweatpants, winter jacket, gloves, three pairs of sweat socks, and no shoes. While most people would be sweating heavily under these circumstances, I was ice cold and shivering. I was fighting to gain control of my movements, so that I could control the car. I closed all the windows and turned the heat up all the way. I miraculously made it to the hospital without killing myself or anyone else.

When I arrived I pulled up to the front door and started to get out of my car. The guard tried to stop me from leaving my car there but after taking one look at me he backed off and I stumbled through the front doors, getting strange looks from everyone around. No one made a move to assist me in any way. I think they were too frightened by my countenance. Fortunately, the elevator was on the main floor and as soon as I pushed the button the doors opened. When they opened again, I literally fell out of the elevator. Two P.A.'s and two nurses were waiting for me with a wheelchair. They picked me up, put me in the wheelchair, and rushed me to an empty room. They helped me sit on top of the blower vent in the room and I turned the air conditioning off and turned the heat on full blast. They couldn't believe what they were seeing! They were sweating from the heat and I was freezing. Dr.

Kenyon had called after I left the house and Lynne told him what was going on and that I was en route to the hospital. He had given them instructions to start an I.V. with a drug that he thought would stop or at least slow down the chills. They couldn't get the hooded sweatshirt off because I was still shaking so badly, so they finally just cut the sleeve open. They tried to get the needle into a vein, failing twice because I was shaking so much. They got me off the vent and on the bed and, while two P.A.'s held me still, the nurse got the needle in the vein and got the I.V. going. I wanted as many blankets as they could find. Nurses were running in with blankets and piling them on top of me. Fourteen blankets later I was still shaking and freezing. They tried taking my temperature several times but I was chattering so much I almost broke the thermometer. After an hour of this the chills subsided and everyone started to relax. By then the room was filled with P.A.'s and nurses, not believing what they were seeing. I told them to start getting ice packs ready and why.

I guess they didn't believe me because no one did anything. I started shedding the blankets, gloves, sweat suit, socks, until I had nothing on except my shorts. I began to sweat. This time the heat was turned off and the air conditioner was turned on full blast. My temperature soon hit 106 degrees and the ice packs were arriving fast now. They were put behind my head, on my forehead, on both sides of my neck, under both arms, and in my groin. In other words near all the lymphatic drainage sites. The fever was always easier for me to handle than the chills and I was able to keep up a conversation with the people in the room. The fever lasted for about an hour and a half and then subsided. When my temperature was down to 100 degrees I said I wanted to return home. Dr. Kenyon had been checking in frequently and he said that if I was feeling that much better I could go home. However, they wouldn't let me drive. Not only was it too dangerous for me but their liability would be too great. One of the male nurses drove me home in my car and another followed to take him back to the hospital.

Lynne had also been checking in with the hospital frequently and was aware of what was going on and what had happened. When I returned home she was upset but under control. We discussed what had gone on and decided that, if the side effects were strong enough to overpower the morphine and were getting worse each day instead of better, it meant that things were getting out of control and we would have to re-evaluate the whole treatment. I told all this to Dr. Kenyon that night on the phone. I asked him to call Houston in the morning and bring them up-to-date on what had been happening and to find out what direction we should go from here. I kept thinking that the C-Parvum must be having some sort of effect on the cancer because the side effects kept getting worse. I was also worried that they were having some sort of deleterious effect upon everything else in my body too and I wasn't sure how much longer I could take this.

Dr. Kenyon called Houston, but Dr. Fredericks was out of town for the day and no one else there was familiar enough with my case to guide us. I also called Houston because I wanted to know firsthand what was going on and why. When I found out Dr. Fredericks was out of town I spoke with Madeline; she told me something was wrong and I had better get in touch with Dr. Fredericks as soon as possible.

After working for four hours the next day I reported in at three at the hospital, not thinking I was going to take another treatment until we heard from Houston. Dr. Kenyon told me that Dr. Fredericks was out of town until the next day. I didn't tell him that I had also called because I didn't see any point in it at that time. We discussed the previous night and decided that since the morphine didn't block the side effects it might have enhanced them. We decided to try it again, one last time, without the morphine. It was like an instant replay of the previous night. The incredible chills, the mad dash to the hospital, except with a friend driving me this time, the high fever, blankets, ice packs. After that I told Dr. Kenyon that was the end of the treatments until we got clarification from Houston about what was going on and why.

I also decided to call Dr. Fredericks and reached him just after he had spoken with Dr. Kenyon. He believed that since the morphine wasn't working it would indeed be dangerous for me to continue with the C-Parvum and therefore said that we should discontinue its use immediately. He did want me to start the chemotherapy in two days after I had had time to rest from the ordeal of the C-Parvum. After nine days of misery, I felt like a newly released prisoner. Just knowing that I was off the C-Parvum gave me a great feeling. Lynne and I went out to dinner with some friends that night, and I finally got a good night's sleep.

Looking back on the original episode of C-Parvum under Dr. Norom, it was still the prevailing opinion that I had received an overdose of the drug. The side effects lasted well over thirty hours and were on a continuous cycle, while the side effects under Dr. Kenyon lasted six to eight hours, maximum, and, once over, were over for good until I received another treatment.

After the two-day rest period I was ready to start the chemotherapy. Dr. Kenyon was a little concerned about the chemotherapy because I seemed to react in such strange ways to different drugs. He had never seen anyone walk away from a dose of morphine the way I did, in addition to the strange reactions I had to the C-Parvum. He was very familiar with the DTIC and the Actinomycin D and their side effects but had never seen them given one on top of the other. He was concerned about my possible reaction to this combination of drugs. He preferred hospitalizing me for the first five-day period so they could monitor what was happening and have some idea what to expect during this portion of my treatment. After I checked into the hospital, Dr. Kenyon explained that he wanted to sedate me in an attempt to minimize the side effects, which he expected to be quite severe since the drugs were given one immediately after the other, and each one on its own has severe side effects. I was expecting to lose all my hair and quite a bit of weight and be totally miserable during the course of the chemotherapy.

An hour after the sedative was administered, I felt no effect at all and Dr. Kenyon decided to try again. The next dose was given through the I.V. tube that was established in order to give the chemotherapy. He was *sure* I would get drowsy this time. Half an hour later he walked in and there I was, sitting up watching television and playing solitaire. Dr. Kenyon laughingly said, "I'll fix your wagon now." He didn't want to put me completely out because that could prove dangerous while on chemotherapy, but he did want me getting sleepy and groggy. He succeeded this time and I was between sleep and drowsiness when the first dose of the chemicals was given. I remember hearing people whispering around me and a burning sensation in my arm at the I.V. site. An hour and a half later I came awake *fast*. I started vomiting violently and didn't stop for almost five hours. This continued for the next few days. The chemotherapy side effects were supposed to diminish each day until the fourth or fifth day, when there should just be a queasy feeling with little or no vomiting at all. With me each day was exactly like the one before it. The fifth day was just as violent as the first. After the initial five-day treatment I waited the seventeen-day interim period and returned for the next five days of chemotherapy. This visit was exactly the same as the first.

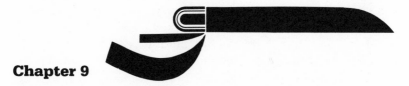

Chapter 9

I had heard bits of information about the use of marijuana during chemotherapy to alleviate the severe side effects. It supposedly lessened the nausea to a great degree, but perhaps the most important thing is that it helps the patients to retain or increase their appetites. It's very important to maintain good nutrition during chemotherapy because your body needs it more than ever. However, because there were no studies at that time on the use of marijuana, there was very little literature about it. I encountered what I felt was my first solid evidence on a television show. Several cancer patients in New Mexico who were currently on chemotherapy were interviewed. They verified that in their cases the marijuana did indeed counteract the adverse reactions and made chemotherapy almost bearable. I started asking every doctor I could find about this and they unanimously agreed: to their knowledge there were no studies available and thus no benefits to be derived from marijuana and they would recommend against its usage. That didn't make any sense at all to me. Simply because there were no studies done on it doesn't mean there weren't any benefits from it. The interview with the cancer patients weighed very heavily on my mind and to me that was worth all the studies in the world. If you haven't guessed by now, I am more than a little stubborn and not one to simply give in on something like this. I decided to try it anyway. While I had some past experience in smoking cigarettes, although I had quit five years prior, I did not know the first thing about how to smoke pot. I did have a friend who had experimented with it before and showed me the technique.

For the third five-day treatment period I was an outpatient. Lynne would drop me off at the hospital and then return in an hour or so to pick me up. We went right home and I would go upstairs onto the outside back balcony, sit down, and smoke a joint. Amazingly enough, it worked. I didn't vomit once. I didn't feel all that great either, but it was a big improvement over the other two chemotherapy periods. I continued the marijuana usage throughout my chemotherapy. I never told any of my doctors what I was doing though. It is interesting that in the last few years studies have been popping up about the effectiveness of marijuana in stopping the side effects of chemotherapy, and in the treatment of glaucoma. A few states, such as Florida and New Mexico, have legalized it for medical purposes and it can be obtained in pill form with the proper prescriptions. Unfortunately, from all I have read to date, the pill is not nearly as effective as smoking a high-quality marijuana joint. While there is now little doubt that marijuana is

successful in overcoming the side effects of chemotherapy **61**
without interfering with its effectiveness, it's the long-term
side effects, if any, that remain unknown. I want to relate a
story here that is 100 percent true. There was a girl in Grand
Rapids, Michigan, who had leukemia. She was dying and for
some reason the doctors were still pumping her full of chemotherapy. She was miserable. She had several brothers and sis-
ters in college who began giving her marijuana, with her parents' permission. It did indeed make her ordeal more bearable.
In fact, she testified before a Michigan legislative committee
on the use of marijuana for cancer patients and in the treatment of glaucoma. In spite of the illegality of marijuana, and
with her parents' continued support, she stated she would
continue using the drug. It made her suffering more bearable
for her and, because of that, for her family as well. She died
shortly after testifying. The point of this story is that, even
with the scarcity of evidence regarding long-term usage of
marijuana, most cancer patients on chemotherapy are more
concerned about just making it through to the next day and if
there is something that will make life a little more bearable
there is no excuse for not permitting it. To date I do not believe there is any evidence at all that says marijuana is addic-
tive; therefore, why hasn't it been approved for use by cancer
patients on chemotherapy everywhere. I am very bitter about
the fact that most state legislatures and the U.S. Congress are
dragging their feet and not doing what should be done to
lessen the pain and suffering that could at least be alleviated if
not obliterated.

However, cancer patients, as a whole, do not have the political organization or the clout to influence the politicians. To
further exemplify this, let's go back to the girl in Michigan
who testified before the legislative committee. A lot of media
coverage was given to that and the legislature approved over-
whelmingly to legalize the use of marijuana for cancer and
glaucoma patients. Funny thing though, several years later it
has still not gotten final approval. In essence, the lobbyists
who were against its use have gotten it tied up somewhere
and again politics is standing in the way of something that

could make life a little more bearable for many people on chemotherapy. I do congratulate the states that have approved its use for having the intelligence, the foresight, and the compassion to approve such measures. I would also like to point out that I have spoken with several other cancer patients who tried marijuana while on chemotherapy and they, like me, have never touched the stuff after they were taken off chemotherapy.

There is another controversy going on currently, concerning the use of heroin for cancer patients who are dying and are in intractable pain. Because of the fear of addiction this has not been approved and I find that deplorable. How can people say they are afraid of patients becoming addicted to something that they will probably not live long enough to become addicted to but that would just make their last days more bearable.

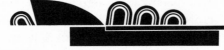

Chapter 10

Chemotherapy is actually an immunodepressant. In other words, it depresses the body's immunologic system and restricts the natural defenses from fighting off not only the cancer, which it obviously wasn't doing a very good job of anyway, but also everything else. The chemotherapy is supposed to battle the cancer-causing cells, but in the process it kills the healthy cells it comes in contact with too, causing the patient to become even weaker than before. Rather than depressing the body's natural defense system it would seem to make more sense to stimulate it and get the body to fend off the cancer cells and to at least help in its own defense. We should build up the immunologic system and support and encourage it rather than tear it down. With the possible exception of certain leukemias where chemotherapy has proved very effective, I believe that the current applications are another step in the march to finding a cure but that in their present form will not be around very much longer. In a conversation that I had with Dr. Kenyon, and this was long after I had been off the chemotherapy, he said he was not sure but that almost as many people had been hurt by chemotherapy as had been helped, simply because of its weakening effects, both mental and physical.

Near the end of September, before starting another course of the chemotherapy, I was scheduled to return to Houston for testing and evaluation. Ten days before I was to leave, a bluish-looking spot appeared on my neck where I had had the radical neck dissection. I called Dr. Abrams and told him what had happened and he said to come over to his office at once. I could tell that he was upset. After seeing it he said that he wanted to biopsy it as soon as possible. He performed the biopsy the next day. It came back from pathology as meta-static malignant melanoma. I knew from my readings that metastatic meant *spreading*. I said, "Great, just great! After all the ———— surgery, immunotherapy, and chemotherapy, here I am, right back to square one!" Dr. Abrams said that it could just be an errant cell that was left behind from the surgery and had started to grow again. He was hedging a little, but I wasn't sure why. I didn't find out until months later that he was afraid this was the beginning of a very rapid decline for me, ultimately leading to my death. It had been his experi-ence, as it had with most doctors, that once the spots start appearing the patient usually dies within a three- or four-month period. I returned to Dr. Abrams the next week to have the stitches removed from the biopsy and showed him another spot that had suddenly appeared about two inches from the one he had just removed. Because I was going to Houston in a few days he preferred I show it to them. He called and informed Dr. Fredericks of the situation prior to my arrival.

Dr. Fredericks took one look at it and said that he had no doubt about what it was but wanted to have it removed imme-diately anyway for confirmation. As expected, it was meta-static malignant melanoma. Dr. Fredericks said that individual spots by themselves were not all that significant as long as they were confined to the surgery site and that Dr. Abrams had been correct in stating they could just be errant cells left over from the surgery. These microscopic cells, invisible to the naked eye, may have been in droplets of blood that became caught in the surgery site and worked their way to the surface as they were growing. However, the appearance of the spots was an indication that the chemotherapy wasn't working either and Dr. Fredericks decided to discontinue it. We discussed all the reactions that I had had to the C-Parvum and the chemotherapy and he said that it didn't make any sense to continue with something that obviously wasn't working. He explained that in the past the standard way of treating melanoma was with the use of BCG (bacillus Calmette-Guérin, a tuberculosis vaccine), but that through the years it had proven ineffective and its use had been discontinued. However, it was an immunologic stimulant and with the very strange way that I was reacting to the drugs I was on he felt that it was worth a try to see if it couldn't at least stimulate my immunologic system a little. We decided to give it a try.

I returned home and called Dr. Kenyon. I told him what Dr. Fredericks had suggested and we started on the BCG the following day. BCG is given by first drawing, with a needle, a grid on an area of the body about four inches by four inches and then pouring the BCG solution over the area and letting it absorb into the tissue through the grid. Dr. Kenyon administered the first treatment. I was to have one treatment per week. The side effects from the drug were supposed to be minimal—a slightly elevated fever, slight achiness, and so on. I never had any side effects at all. The next week I arrived on schedule for my treatment and it was administered by one of the P.A.'s. I thought that it felt a little heavy-handed but decided to just grin and bear it. I bit down on the pillow as I was lying on my stomach while he was working on my back. After leaving, I stopped in at a convenience store to get a cup of coffee. As I was walking out, the girl behind the counter squealed as if frightened and I turned to see what had happened. She said there was blood all over the back of my shirt. I knew what it had to be, so I returned to the hospital and Dr. Kenyon looked at it. Sure enough, the P.A. had cut through the skin completely and I was bleeding all over the place. No wonder the procedure had hurt like hell. That, needless to say, was the last time that individual ever administered the BCG.

I remained on the BCG once a week for the ninety-day period between trips to Houston. On December 11, 1978, I returned to Houston for further testing and evaluation. I had received seven treatments and had undergone the appearance and removal of several new spots. The one serious difference in the appearance of the most recent spots was that they had been on my right arm and right shoulder. All the previous spots had appeared on the left side of my neck, where the radical neck surgery had been performed. Dr. Fredericks explained that the human body has an imaginary line down the center that separates the immunological system and that nothing can cross that line left to right or right to left without first going through the heart, liver, lungs, or brain. He said that this was the most serious development to date and that it made no sense at all to continue with this treatment, which obviously wasn't working either, and that there really wasn't anything further that could be done. In his opinion, and I guess it's only natural that I remember his exact words, "Since you're young, strong, and obviously a fighter, I would say one year, possibly two, maybe a little longer, but probably a whole lot less." He thought it advisable to get all my affairs in order and to make all the necessary arrangements. I had been told several times before that I was a terminal case, but this was the first time that I was told outright that I was going to die and fairly soon and that's it!

Afterward I walked over to Rice University, which is only a few blocks away, and walked around the very pleasant, beautiful campus for a while just thinking. No tears, no hysteria, just thinking about what I should do at this point. I decided that it would serve no purpose at all to call anyone long distance and it would serve no purpose to tell anyone anything until I at least had had a chance to figure out what direction I wanted to go from this point. I left Rice and went back to the hospital to see Madeline. She told me that she had already heard and that she was sorry. I jokingly asked her if this changed my category. She said I had now reached the top of the scale, that there was only one higher level, which was jokingly referred to as level five. I asked what level five was and she said dead. We both laughed, but only because it was better than crying. She wished me luck and said to keep up the fight, that at this point the most important thing for me was to maintain a positive mental attitude. That night I went out to dinner with Harry and Mary, the Champion sales representative and his wife in the Houston area, and really had an enjoyable time. I never told them what had happened that day. I saw no reason to. I also figured that there would be no better way to ruin an evening than to tell someone you had just been told there was nothing further anyone could do to help save your life. I needed a little time away from that.

I returned home deciding not to tell anyone yet. Lynne was starting to have a difficult time handling all the things that were happening with the appearance of the spots and was starting to take a very negative attitude. I am not sure if I decided not to tell her to protect her or myself, but in any case I didn't feel that this was the proper time to tell her. I was also learning not to tell anything I didn't want her to know to anyone who knew her, because it inevitably got back to her immediately. However, I did tell the two other Champion sales reps in the state, who are just like brothers to me. I told them what had transpired and that I was getting my affairs in order and was starting to make my final preparations. I also told them *not* to tell anyone at all, especially no one in Champion. I did not want them to have this information yet. After discussing it with them, I surprisingly felt quite a bit better.

Drs. Kenyon and Abrams were the only others who were aware of my situation. Dr. Abrams gets annoyed when there are time limits placed on people. He is fond of saying that doctors are not gods and cannot predict when someone is going to die. In Dr. Fredericks' defense, I told Dr. Abrams that I pushed him into giving me his opinion and his prognosis. Dr. Abrams also told me to try to keep a positive attitude, because it was the most important thing that I had going for me at that point. Dr. Kenyon, on the other hand, wasn't at all sure that he agreed with the diagnosis. He believed there seemed to be something within me working in my favor because the spots kept coming to the surface and nothing had invaded any major organ; he thought I was fighting this off on my own. It was his opinion that this process could continue as it was for years. As soon as a spot appeared we would remove it in order to keep the cancer cell population as low as possible and not let anything we were aware of get better established.

I made an appointment with the rabbi and the cantor and told them of the situation and that I wanted to start making preparations for my funeral. I felt that the worst time to make plans for a funeral was after someone had died. I wanted to remove this burden from my family and make sure that it was done in a financially responsible way. We worked everything out and the cantor called the funeral home and set up an appointment for me with the funeral director. I learned that you even get a 10 percent discount when you pay for a funeral in advance. For some reason I think that's pretty funny. Just think, maybe soon we will be able to clip a coupon from the evening paper for a sale on funerals over the weekend.

My next stop was to meet with my attorney to make sure my will was updated. We set up a trust for Lynne and Jared. I wanted the assurance of knowing that after I was gone they would be well provided for. After doing all this I felt better about everything. I didn't want to leave any loose ends and it was important to me to know that everything had been taken care of in the manner that I wanted and that Lynne and Jared would always be financially secure. It was bothering me quite a bit, however, that I still had not told Lynne what was happening. She was still taking a negative route though, and the more I thought about telling her the more I felt it would only make things worse for all of us. I decided just to keep things quiet for a little while longer.

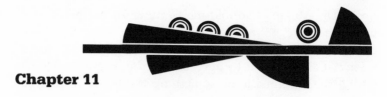

Chapter 11

Before he performed the radical neck dissection, Dr. Abrams had told me that I would probably lose some of the mobility in my left shoulder. I wouldn't be able to raise my left arm above my shoulder and I would have very little strength in it, because of all the muscles that were being taken out of the neck and shoulder area. I wasn't really upset about it at the time because there was nothing I could do about it. I would just have to deal with it and make the best of the situation.

As soon as I was allowed to get out of bed I began exercising. I would walk around the entire fourth floor of the hospital, working up to as rapid a pace as I could. Then I added going up and down the flights of stairs in the exit stairwells. There are eight floors in the hospital and I would go up and down all eight floors several times in the morning, again in the afternoon, and again after visiting hours at night.

When Dr. Abrams released me from the hospital I returned to work the next day and started exercising that same day. Dr. Abrams learned to let me do what I could because he knew that I was going to anyway. I started swimming immediately, because not only did swimming exercise the very areas I wanted to work on, but the water gave support to those areas as well. I started working on the weight machines and after one week I started jogging again. I exercised every day regardless of the weather conditions. I jogged outside every day no matter what. If it was ninety degrees I ran, if it was minus ten I ran, if it snowed I ran, if it rained I ran, if it was sunny I ran. In the winter I would often come in with frozen-solid eyebrows. Obviously, I swam inside, but I swam every day and worked on the weight machines at least four times a week.

I quickly learned that I couldn't play tennis right away. I had lost all control of tossing with my left arm, so I couldn't serve.

After about a year of exercising on all the other things, I was able to return slowly to tennis until I could toss the ball as well as I ever did. There are still a few movements that I have difficulty with, but nothing that I haven't been able to work around.

I was not going to be denied any of the exercise that I have always loved. I have always believed that if I were willing to put in the time and worked hard enough there was nothing that I couldn't overcome as far as physical limitations from any surgery that I have had or will have in connection with the cancer. Exercise has always been more than just physical conditioning to me. It has done as much if not more for my mental state as my physical state. It has been an escape, a way to work out frustrations and feelings of anger. I have worked and worked and worked to regain full use of my left arm and I have succeeded. I still get some very strange looks at the athletic club because of my large and ominous-looking scars. However, for the most part, I don't mind anymore, because I have learned to live with my body the way it is. I really don't have any other choice in the matter—I can't trade it in.

The athletic club that I go to has been a godsend to me. I would go there after a night on the C-Parvum and just sit in the sauna or jog or swim a little and it would seem like the C-Parvum was just a bad dream and nothing for me to be concerned about. The people who worked there were great too. I don't know if they were aware that I had cancer, but when I came dragging in there with my tie open they would usually refrain from any business, even though they were also customers of mine.

Now that I was no longer receiving any treatments, I was desperate to get back into some sort of "normal" life style. I still had to have blood tests once a month and X rays every other month, but aside from that I was like everybody else. I quickly returned to a daily routine of work and exercise.

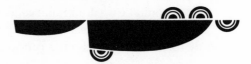

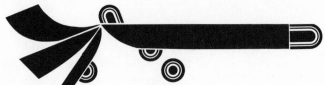

Chapter 12

My biggest problem was my family. Lynne couldn't handle the total uncertainty of what was going on and she was starting to destroy not only our relationship but also herself in the process. I tried several times to talk with her about it, yet she seemed unable to sit down and discuss it rationally for any length of time. Whenever I would bring it up her first reaction would be, "What's the matter, something has happened, hasn't it, there's something wrong, I can tell it." Despite my reassurances that nothing was wrong, she would still get upset. I tried to be as understanding and gentle with her as I could, but it was getting more and more difficult every day. She finally broke down and told me that she was sick of it, couldn't handle it, and didn't want to hear about it anymore. In fact she implied that if the spots kept appearing, indicating to her that I would die soon, she would have to leave because she was not prepared to deal with that. It was, perhaps, the first time that Lynne was completely honest with me and with herself about the situation. I not only understood what she was saying and why, but I appreciated her leveling with me. At least we both knew where we stood. I know she is mad at me for having cancer and very resentful and bitter at the world for putting this burden on her shoulders. She needs to find a way to express herself and yet even after talking with her friends she still is very angry and bitter that it is she who is in this situation and not someone else. I imagine that Lynne's feelings are quite normal for someone in this predicament. However, those feelings make the total situation even more of a problem for me. I have to contend not only with the disease process but also the problems that it presents to my family. There should be no doubt that cancer brings with it more than just a disease. It brings many, many nonmedical problems not only for the person who has cancer but for the family as well.

Those problems are real and should not be ignored; they **71**
must be dealt with.

There are times when I get mad as hell at Lynne because
she has not been able to cope with my cancer in the same
manner that I have. That's not fair to her and I realize it. She
faces a different set of problems than I do and she is scared.
She is a very loving, caring, and warm person. Perhaps sometimes I lose track of that. Perhaps I am overly critical and
show a lack of understanding of the position she is in. Everyone feels very sorry for Lynne because of the difficult situation she is in—just as I feel sorry for the spouses as well as
the individuals with cancer in the cases that I as a third party
have seen. However, when you are one of the parties involved,
your perspective is totally different. The pressure on both
sides is enormous, especially when the viewpoints are different. Each one feels that the pressure on him or her is greater
than on the other. In our case I am concerned about not just
staying alive, but living a quality life (without pain, able to
function in the world as an independent person without the
constant aid of someone else to do this or that for me, to be
able to do for myself—I never want to be kept alive by machines); about being able to support my family; about being
able to be the role model for my son that I want to be; about
being able to be a contributing, productive individual in our
society; and, finally, about not having to go through a linger-
ing death. If and when I do have to die I want it to be as quick
and as painless as possible.

Lynne's position is quite different from mine. She worries
about being a single parent, about handling the finances when
she is on her own, about having total responsibility for herself
and Jared, about being an independent unmarried woman in
a world that she is not sure she can handle without a spouse.
She feels that my problems end when I die but hers continue
in a different way and, therefore, she carries the larger burden. I don't think there is a person in the world who can find
either of us wrong or unreasonable in our concerns and fears.
On the other hand, in a situation such as this the parties involved cannot afford to let sympathy and pity creep into their

feelings. I cannot afford to fall into the bottomless pit of self-pity as it would detract from my primary goal of staying alive in the manner in which I want. I don't want Lynne feeling sorry for me as I need her there to make sure that I don't lose track of my primary goal. Neither can I let myself feel sorry for Lynne and Jared and let that affect my better judgment so that I might do something simply because I feel sorry for them now that might have a negative effect later on.

The two things that both Lynne and Jared need in their lives more than anything else are security and stability, and these are the two things that I cannot give them or myself. I am doing my best to make sure they will always be secure in a financial sense but this by itself has caused more insecurities for all of us. I don't know what is going to happen from one day to the next in my life and this is perhaps the worst way for Lynne to live. I wish I could tell her that I will be fine tomorrow but I can't, just as no doctor can tell me that. I have heard a thousand times that none of us knows what tomorrow is going to bring and that's nice to say when everything is fine today, but when everything is not fine today and you don't know *if* there is a future, it makes for a very difficult life.

Lynne is a teacher. Not *just* a teacher, a *great* teacher. She teaches English to gifted seventh graders. She relates to them in such a way that they really love her class and look forward to it each day even though she gives them a great deal of work to do and is very demanding of them. She challenges them and they do the same for her. It is truly a fascinating thing to see. Watching her teach is like seeing a great performance on stage. She holds her students' attention and you can just see them soaking it all in. Her job has been one of the best things in her life, especially since I contracted cancer. It gives her a way of escaping into her world that she enjoys, and without that I doubt she would have made it this far. She needs it and she has put a lot into it. It has been as good for her as she has been for it. She gets very close to most of her students and if one of them has a problem it's almost as if it were her own problem. She has always had a very Pollyanna-type outlook on life. I don't mean that in a derogatory way either. It was one of the things that attracted me to her when we were in college. She is a very bubbly, warm, friendly individual, much more so than I. I think that she expects too much from people though. She expects them to treat her in the same manner in which she usually treats them, and when they don't, she gets upset. Unfortunately, Lynne also thinks that her problems are everyone else's too, and that's just not the way it is. Because everyone else in the world is not experiencing the same hardships she is, she has become very intolerant of others' problems. No one's problems are as big as hers in her mind. I wish I could sit her down and ease her fears about what has been happening in our lives, but to date I just haven't been able to find the way to do that.

The next spot appeared in the first week of March 1979, right on schedule. There seemed to be a ninety-day pattern in the appearance of the spots now. It was a curious phenomenon to everyone, but no one understood why. They would always appear subcutaneously (under the skin) and this was even stranger. I didn't tell Lynne about the new spot. I called Dr. Abrams and told him and he scheduled the surgery for the following day. I wasn't sure how to tell Lynne, or if I should tell her at all. I decided to tell her before the surgery but waited until the following morning. I told her about it very casually while reassuring her that this was no different than any of the others and there was nothing to worry about. She was upset about the appearance of the spot and the fact that I hadn't told her. Now, instead of wanting to be in the dark about my condition, she wanted to know everything and had begun questioning me frequently about what my progress or symptom development was. Before I returned to Dr. Abrams' office for removal of the sutures, another spot appeared. This one was removed two days later and again another spot appeared before I had the sutures removed from the previous incision. This was getting to be sort of a ritual. I was almost as at home in the operating room as the doctors and nurses were and I was getting to know the procedures and personnel by heart.

After Dr. Abrams removes a spot we both look at it in the

operating room and can usually tell by its appearance if it is malignant, even before the pathology report. This recent episode was the one time that Dr. Abrams would tell me he thought the events were serious enough for me to make sure all my affairs were in order. He said the appearance of so many spots so rapidly was perhaps the most ominous sign of all. I saw Dr. Kenyon the next day and he said the same thing. I was leaving for Houston again in a few days and both Dr. Abrams and Dr. Kenyon informed Dr. Fredericks of these developments prior to my arrival. I had decided not to share this news with Lynne at least until after I returned from Houston and I heard what they had to say about the situation.

Unfortunately, Dr. Fredericks said about the same thing: "Mr. Shapiro, nothing has changed, the disease is progressing and there's nothing we can do to stop it; it's just a matter of time. The rush of spots all at close intervals signals the end." He told me that the major organ it would hit most probably would be the liver, but sometimes it hits the lungs or brain first. It is relatively rare for it to metastasize to the heart. Perhaps because I was hearing it so often, I seemed to take the news that I was dying in stride and didn't let it upset me. I don't want to imply that I was elated either, but there was something very strange at work here. Here I am, supposedly dying and I don't feel bad, nor have I ever felt bad. I don't mean emotionally because no matter who you are when you are told you are dying you feel bad emotionally. I mean physically. I didn't then, nor do I now, feel physically bad. That being the case, I have always found it very hard to accept the fact that I am supposed to be dying, and my gut reaction was, no I am not dying. How can I be so close to death and not feel bad? I know what the medical facts are and I can't deny them, yet I also know how I feel and I can't deny that either. I was well aware that mental attitude plays a very large, albeit unexplainable, role, and I believed that if I gave in at that time I really would die but if I kept going the way I was then I was not going to die. I was actually getting a little mad about it because I resented the fact that I was told I was going to die while I was still feeling physically excellent. Maybe it's be-

cause I didn't understand the course that melanoma follows, **75**
but I wasn't about to just agree and die. I was ready to fight.

After I had seen Dr. Fredericks, my Houston associate, Harry, had arranged a personal tour of the NASA space center and it was just what I needed; I was completely fascinated. It not only got my mind off cancer for awhile but I got excited about what I was seeing and hearing; I loved it. It was something I will remember for the rest of my life. One of the astronauts gave us the tour. He showed us the space shuttle and we were permitted to stay while they ran a test landing. It was fascinating. We also saw a mock-up of Skylab. This was during the time there was so much publicity about Skylab coming down. He showed us the pieces they thought would be the ones returning to earth and where they thought they would land; as it turned out he was amazingly accurate. We met several of the other astronauts and support personnel and they were all very interesting people.

Harry, his wife, Mary, and I went out to dinner that night and I again thoroughly enjoyed myself. They are both very gracious people and have been exceptionally nice to me. I again didn't share the medical news of that day with them; I saw no reason to get them upset. Just being with people you know and like at times like that, whether they are aware of the facts or not, makes a big difference. It is impossible to express how much I appreciate their being there at a time I needed a friendly, comfortable atmosphere. Thanks, Mary and Harry.

I returned home still wondering what, if anything, to tell Lynne. How could I tell her something that I myself had trouble believing? In spite of the clinical evidence, I was still unwilling to accept the fact I was dying. I was not dying, I was living, and I was returning home to live not die. With that in mind what was I supposed to tell Lynne? I couldn't tell her that the doctors thought I was in the final stages of the disease and about to die but I didn't believe it. She was nervous enough about things and that would drive her crazy. Neither could I completely lie and tell her nothing at all because she knew about the spots. Therefore I told her that there really wasn't anything to be concerned about, that these spots were the same as all the rest and we shouldn't get overly worried about them.

After returning home I got together with the two other Champion sales reps and I explained what was going on. I told them that even though I didn't believe it I had to make sure I was prepared for anything and couldn't afford to have any loose ends. I also told them that I didn't want this information to go any further, especially not back to the home office. We had made plans to get together with our families the following weekend and we had a nice time together. However, one of the wives happened to mention to Lynne that I had been told I only had a year left to live and that if there was anything they could do to help just to call. Lynne didn't say anything about it until the next day. She was acting very strange and I had no idea why. She must have spent most of that day on the phone with Dr. Abrams, Dr. Kenyon, and Dr. Johnson; in fact, she went in to see Dr. Johnson and spoke with him personally. They all reiterated what I had been told in Houston the previous two trips there.

Several things upset me about this incident. First, Lynne found out about the things I had been keeping from her, although I guess that was bound to happen sooner or later. Second, the abrupt manner in which she found out was too hard on her. Third, since Lynne and I had become friends with Dr. Kenyon and his wife, we were seeing them socially, too. I began discovering that things I had discussed with Dr. Kenyon and thought were being kept between the two of us were getting back to his wife, who then was telling Lynne. I told Dr. Kenyon what had been happening and that Lynne was getting to be a problem. He promised to keep things just between the two of us from that point on. Lynne now knew what the actual story was and I waited for her to take the next step. It has definitely been very difficult for her and she has had a hard time coping with the situation but she has been trying as best she can.

While in Houston I had discussed with Dr. Fredericks the problem I was having at home. He was very compassionate about it and said two things. First, it wasn't an uncommon occurrence in marriages where one partner had cancer. Second, **77** he thought I should speak with the psychologist and social workers at M. D. Anderson. They are very familiar with this problem and could possibly be of some help. They too said it was a very common problem among families of cancer patients and is why the divorce rate is higher than normal among these families. This is especially true when the person with cancer is capable of living a relatively normal life, like I was. They suggested that I try to be honest with her, tell her how I felt, and see if she would get professional help, adding that I should probably go with her. I explained all this to Lynne and she agreed, but she wanted to choose the doctor herself. I told her I was willing to see the doctor with her or see him or her privately if she wanted me to. Lynne agreed to this also. However, after not hearing anything for a month, I asked her if she had seen anyone. She said, "No," adding that she hadn't had the time, but that she would do it. Another month passed and I asked her again and she said, "No," again giving the same reason as before. This time I told her to do it or I was leaving. She came home one day and said she had seen someone and she thought it was useless. I suggested she try someone else. I asked her if she had been totally honest with the person she had seen and she said, "No." After only one visit, she wasn't being fair in saying the doctor was useless, especially if she hadn't put all her cards on the table. She said she would see him again, and she did return but with the same results as the first time.

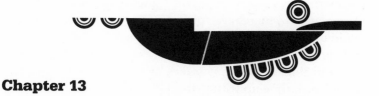

Chapter 13

I was getting ready to return to Houston for my ninety-day checkup and, as if on schedule, a spot appeared. I called Dr. Abrams and he scheduled the surgery. By this time I had discovered so many spots that Dr. Abrams didn't require me to come to the office to confirm them; he would just schedule the surgery and see it for the first time in the operating room. He trusted my judgment and his trust was more than justified as I found every spot almost as soon as it appeared. We always talk a lot in the operating room about any number of topics. Since all the spots are removed with only a local anesthetic, I am wide awake. This time I told Dr. Abrams I couldn't justify in my own mind that here I was, supposedly dying and yet I felt great. There was obviously cancer still present, because we were cutting it out. I was sure more spots would appear, but nothing seemed to be happening. He said he was curious about the same thing but didn't have any explanations for it. There definitely seems to be some sort of pattern to the appearance of the spots now, but nothing else seems to follow, and that is very strange.

I returned to Houston on June 19, 1979, and again Dr. Fredericks told me that it was just a matter of time, although I seemed to be doing amazingly well in the face of some very stiff odds. We discussed why the spots were appearing subcutaneously and had not internalized to one of the major organs. He didn't have a ready answer for that. The only thing he could think of was that the internal temperature of my body, especially in the major organs, was too high and the cancer cells couldn't establish themselves and grow in one spot. As they traveled throughout my body and got closer to the surface, the temperature dropped and these cells then found a suitable climate to settle and grow in. As they became bigger and could be seen or felt, I discovered them and they were removed, thereby keeping the cell population down to a minimum. He admitted that this was an off-the-wall theory and I am not sure that anyone really buys it. However, if you stop and think about it, it makes more sense than anything anyone has come up with to this point. I believe that this theory plus my attitude and willingness to fight are the reasons why I am alive right now.

In Houston I again discussed the deteriorating situation at home with the psychologists and social workers at M.D.A. They suggested that maybe I was babying Lynne too much

and was more concerned about how she was doing than how
I was doing. After all, who is the one with cancer? They said it
seemed to be a role reversal. I seemed to be taking it just fine
and Lynne seemed to be coming apart at the seams. They told
me it was going to take a major effort to get Lynne straight-
ened out and that I should make sure she sought out professionals who have experience in this area.

When I returned home from Houston, Lynne agreed to see
another psychologist. One of the problems was to find someone competent in this type of problem. Usually these professionals are found in and around the major medical centers,
not in Lansing, Michigan. She finally decided on one of our
neighbors, who is on the staff at the university. She saw him
several times and seemed to be relating to him very well.
However, since we are neighbors and see each other socially,
he felt it was not in his best interest or Lynne's to continue
because it was too difficult to be objective. Lynne has since
seen three psychologists but none has helped. One of them
even encouraged her to continue her behavior regardless of
the effects it had on me because it was a way for her to vent
her own feelings and it was up to me to deal with it. I am not
sure I follow that logic at all.

Things were getting more and more difficult at home for me
every day. Lynne had started asking me once, twice, five,
sometimes ten times a day if anything had happened, or if
any new spots had appeared. This was getting to be an obses-
sion with her and beginning to get on my nerves. I tried explaining to her that it was getting very difficult to be around
her while she continually gave me the third degree about my
condition, that things were not going to change from one hour
to the next. She kept it up despite my protestations. She would
call Dr. Kenyon or Dr. Abrams just to see if I had been there
without telling her. Whenever it was time for my monthly
blood tests or X rays she would start saying such things as, "I
know they are going to come out bad; I just know that something bad is going to happen." I tried being understanding
and patient, but she finally got to me and I blew up. I told her
that life with cancer was difficult enough without having to

fight her too. If there was ever a time in my life when I needed the support of my family it was certainly a time like this. I said I would not put up with it anymore. I couldn't stand coming home each day because her constant badgering was just getting to be too much for me to take. No matter what I said she always converted it into some sort of disaster. I told her I was leaving. Lynne began crying, saying she didn't know why she behaved that way and promised to stop and to seek help. I felt sorry for her and didn't leave. It hasn't made any difference at all. The only time I have a break from her relentless questioning is when I am away or she has gone to bed at night. That's when I get my work done, work on the book, or just sit and enjoy the peace and quiet. I wasn't just concerned about the effect this was having on me. I was more concerned about the effects it might be having on Jared. What does he think, hearing this stuff every day?

It would be ironical if this book is ever published and gets any degree of attention. Then experts would be coming out of the woodwork saying I did this because of that or I did that because of this. But where are the experts now when I really need them?

I sometimes feel that I am sacrificing myself in order not to hurt those around me. I wish I knew what the right thing to do was, but there is no right or wrong in these situations. Both sides could be argued very successfully. To use Dr. Fredericks' favorite expression, "It is an imponderable." Do I do what's best for me assuming I am going to die within a year or two and deserve a little happiness? Or do I stay put, assuming I am not dying, grin and bear it, try to work things out, and avoid hurting Lynne and Jared by remaining together as a family?

Lynne has taken on a superstitious nature regarding the cancer. She will not use the sheets or towels that were in use at the time of the radical neck surgery. She once left a very expensive pair of suede pants at the cleaners for months and months. I happened to be in the cleaners one day when they mentioned this to me so I picked them up. Lynne said she was afraid to bring those pants back into the house because

something had happened with the cancer the last time she
wore them and she was afraid it would recur if she brought
them back. I have tried and tried to explain to her and the
doctors have all told her: he's doing great, the hell with all the
spots and the reports, he's fighting it off on his own better
than any of the drugs. He feels good and looks good, what
more do you want, what more can you ask for? They have
told her to stop worrying so much and just enjoy life. If I go
on and beat this thing for the next ten years or so, what will
Lynne have to look back on? Nothing but wasted time, and
you can't make that up. You can waste money or many other
things and make it up, but once you've lost time you can *never*
recapture it.

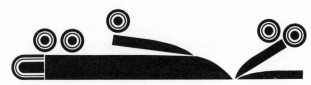

Chapter 14

It was around September of 1979 that I ran across the Elisabeth Kubler-Ross books. I do a lot of work in the library as it is
the only place I can get away from the phone and get some
work done without any interruptions or disturbances. While I
was doing some work there one day, I saw a book that was
obviously out of place. After a few hours I picked it up. It was
Death: The Final Stage of Growth by Elisabeth Kubler-Ross. I
had never heard of the book or the author before, but I opened
it up and started reading. I was fascinated. I finished the book
in the next few days and checked to see what else she had
written. She had written several other books and I read them
all. The others were *On Death and Dying, Questions and Answers on Death and Dying,* and *To Live until We Say Good-Bye.* I
have never been so engrossed, fascinated, and spellbound by
any books.

I would like to see the Kubler-Ross books required reading
for every high school in the country. I can't think of any academic lesson that is more important than what Kubler-Ross

says in her books. These are lessons in life, not death, and can be of more importance to a high school student preparing to embark on a career or academic work than many of the classes they are enrolled in. My doctors had also heard of her and said that she had indeed done some truly amazing work. There are some absolutely incredible parts that I could identify with so readily, not only relating to me because of the cancer but also because of events that occurred when my father or grandparents were dying. I discovered I knew so little about the subject of death and dying and was able to identify some of my experiences and feelings in each of the five stages she described. I think she has opened the closet door on a subject that has been locked away far too long. After all, death is a part of life and we all must face it many times in our lives as those around us die and as we finally confront it ourselves. Dr. Kubler-Ross has shown that death doesn't have to be the cold, frightening thing we often make it out to be. I don't think she has made death an attractive, desirable event, but she has shown us that it can indeed be a beautiful experience. She points out that we should not avoid the subject, especially with the individual who is dying. When persons who are dying want to talk about it, they must be able to talk with someone they feel close to and comfortable with. To prevent this from happening is cruel. Dr. Kubler-Ross says doctors as well as the lay public are afraid of death and often unable to comfort those experiencing it.

After reading the books I can see some of the mistakes I've made. I should have been open and honest about everything and let everyone else worry about handling their own feelings. My brother and my cousin actually are my closest family allies, but the geographical distance between us hinders close, continual communication.

The only way I can continue to successfully fight the cancer is to adopt a somewhat selfish attitude. I must consider what is best for me and what will aid me the most in continuing the fight. This can also be self-defeating. As Kubler-Ross points out, the families of terminally ill people should not have to put up with a lot of abuse from the patient. In my case, specifically, I am saying that the terminally ill person should not have to put up with a lot of abuse from the family. Somehow the belief that whenever there is a tragedy in a family everyone closes ranks and pulls together to overcome the problem may be great in theory but it doesn't always work in reality. People have their own lives to lead, their own families to look after, their own problems to take care of, and in the overly complicated world we live in people cannot always drop everything and help out elsewhere, nor should they be expected to. The world does not wait for anyone to recover from anything, it goes right on by and it is up to you to catch up to it; it will not slow down for you no matter what or who you are. In other words, sometimes you must just take control of things by yourself and do the very best you can to keep up at the same time you are trying to survive. It is commonly called life, and, good or bad, you must live it yourself; no one can do it for you.

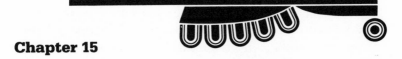

Chapter 15

May 7, 1980: it's five weeks before my next trip to Houston and one week before we are to leave for a short vacation in Las Vegas. Almost on cue, I noticed my neck felt a little sore and stiff in several places. I looked for spots even closer than usual but couldn't find any. However, upon closer examination, I discovered a small lump on the left side of my neck. I went in to see Dr. Abrams but he wasn't sure what it was either. We decided that it should be removed on the assumption that it was a tumor. The surgery was scheduled for May 22, so that I could still go on vacation.

I decided not to tell Lynne until the night before the surgery. I knew this was probably the wrong approach again in the long run, but at the time it was best for me and I didn't need the added problems of telling Lynne at the time.

Wednesday, May 21: when I got home Lynne was just leaving to play tennis and Jared was down the street playing with some friends. I thought, WOW, a little peace and quiet before the storm hits when I tell Lynne about the surgery tomorrow.

She returned an hour and a half later and started right in with, "Something is wrong, I know something is wrong, when are you going in?" She just kept firing the questions at me until I asked her to "calm down, sit down, and let's talk." I casually explained to her that Dr. Abrams and I were going out to lunch the next day and from there we were going to the hospital. He was going to remove a recurrence of the basal cell on my forehead plus a lump on my neck that could be either a fibroma, neuroma, or melanoma. Dr. Abrams was unsure what it was, but there was no need to get upset over this; it was no big deal. It wasn't any different than any of the other times. The basal cell she knew was nothing to worry about and I told her there was at least as good a chance that the lump was a fibroma, or a neuroma, as there was that it was a melanoma. What I didn't tell her was that if it was a melanoma that would mean it was starting to show up in deeper masses than ever before. I explained to her that a neuroma is a ball of nerves that probably resulted from the radical neck surgery when the nerves were cut, and a fibroma was a ball of fatty tissue that formed and was nothing to be concerned about at all. Since it was being done in the outpatient surgery clinic at the university, I would be able to drive myself there and home. She wasn't impressed with my explanations at all and hardly spoke about it for the rest of the night.

Thursday, May 22: I worked all morning and met Dr. Abrams for lunch. I enjoyed this because I got to see a social side of Dr. Abrams that I had not seen before. After lunch we went to the hospital. Dr. Abrams had one other patient to operate on before me. During this time I registered and checked in and got all the preoperation paperwork out of the way. I had been through this enough times to know what lay ahead of me, so I really wasn't too nervous. I read the newspaper while I was waiting. Half an hour later I was taken into the operating room and scrubbed for the surgery. I knew the head nurse

well by now and we kidded around while waiting for Dr.
Abrams. He came into the room, looked at the two areas that
had to be removed, and marked them out. When he finally
got to the lump he was unable to tell right off if it was a malignancy or not. He held it up so that we could examine it; we
both decided it might be a tumor—but it wasn't a malignant
melanoma. It just wasn't the right color.

Every melanoma that has been taken out of me has been
a bluish-black color and this was a healthy pinkish-looking
tissue. Dr. Abrams cut it open to see how it looked on the inside. He thought it was a neuroma, had it marked, and sent it
to the pathologists for analysis, who proclaimed it benign. We
all breathed a little easier at that.

While I was on the table, after the lump was removed, I
chuckled a little to myself. The absurdity of this situation was
hitting me: here I am on the operating table, getting cut up by
the person I had just had lunch with and then examining my
own flesh to see if it was malignant or not and I hadn't lost my
cookies yet. The real test comes with the electric knife though.
You can smell something burning, because it cauterizes the
vessels to stop the bleeding; however, it is different when you
realize that what is burning is you!

I was taken back to my room, got dressed, and left. The
first thing I did when I left was stop at the dairy store on campus and get a chocolate cone. They have great ice cream there
that they make themselves. After that I had several errands to
take care of, including filling a prescription for pain pills, and
then I went home. When I got out of the car I leaned over to
get some packages out of the back seat. I must have popped a
few stitches because I started bleeding all over the place. The
wound in my forehead had opened and it felt like the blood
was just pouring out of me. I grabbed some tissues and went
inside to try to stop the bleeding. Jared had just gotten up
from his nap and was getting ready to go outside to play. I
told the babysitter to take him out front so that he wouldn't be
frightened by all the blood on me and the floor. The babysitter
was frightened and concerned and said she would stay right
in front of the house in case I needed help. I stopped the

bleeding and took a few pain pills. By now the anesthetic was wearing off and my head and neck were pounding in pain. I went out to clean up the blood in the garage so that when Lynne got home she wouldn't think World War III had started. I started bleeding again, went back in the house, and this time laid down for awhile until the bleeding stopped for good. When Lynne got home I took a few more pain pills and started using an ice pack. My forehead, though, felt like someone was standing over me with a sledge hammer trying to separate my head from the rest of my body. I took some stronger pills I had saved from previous operations, but they didn't work either. The ice pack actually helped more than anything else. Finally, about ten o'clock that night, either the pills started working or the pain had subsided enough for me to fall asleep.

During the Memorial Day weekend, Lynne started complaining about how tough things were on her. I finally told her that I was sick and tired of hearing about how tough things were on her, that having cancer wasn't my idea of a good time either. I told her it seemed I was fighting not only the cancer but her too. I understood very well that she had her own set of problems to deal with, but she refused to let anyone help her. I suggested perhaps she should get out and start a new life on her own without the troublesome burden of having a husband with cancer dragging her down. This was said in anger and usually things said in anger should never have been said in the first place. However, in retrospect, at the time I think it shook Lynne up a little that I would call her bluff. I don't think she knew how to handle that. I emphasized to her that under no circumstances would I ever give Jared up but that she was free to leave any time she wished.

She immediately went into my office, picked up the four Kubler-Ross books, which she had steadfastly refused to even look at before, and started reading them. She read the first two that night and the second two the next day (she speed reads at an incredible rate). This was very much out of character for Lynne. She said that she must learn to be independent and rely on herself. She said all of this in such a way it seemed as if I wasn't even there, as if I were dead and buried already. I tried to explain to her that at this time it was a time of optimism, not pessimism, and she just said, "Bullshit, we all know that it is just a matter of time and that no matter what we do it will not work. The truth is that no one knows what the hell to do and they just keep cutting and cutting; maybe we got away this time, but what about the next time, and the time after that?" This attitude, though it only lasted overnight, probably indicates Lynne really does understand what is going on but keeps it suppressed so she doesn't have to face it every day. I was really quite surprised. It also showed that Lynne had some fight in her and I was glad to see that, because if and when anything happens to me, she is going to need every bit of it, in order to build a new life for Jared and herself without me.

Lynne had volunteered to be a collector the next day at a local shopping center for the American Cancer Society by selling flowers. She came home upset that people could be as cold and callous as they are when approached for money. It was her first experience with the fact that, unless something touched them personally, people really don't want to be bothered and can be very cold and abrupt. On the other hand, she did meet some people who wanted to give and wanted to help. Some came up to her and told her of family members who either had cancer presently or had died of cancer. One lady very tearfully gave money, telling Lynne her husband had just died of the disease. So she saw both sides. Some people wanted to help and others (by far the majority) just brushed right on by not wanting to be bothered.

I feel bad for Lynne. I know she desperately wants to do something to help but doesn't know what or how. She doesn't want to lose her husband to cancer and be left alone with a young son to care for. But there is nothing I can do to help her in this instance. Sometimes there are things we must learn for ourselves and I think that this is one of them.

Thursday, May 29: I returned to Dr. Abrams' office to have the stitches removed. The previous evening I had noticed a very tiny lump on my right temple, right above the area where the melanoma had been removed several months ago. Dr. Abrams wanted me to keep track of it and show it to Dr. Fredericks when I got to Houston in three weeks.

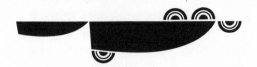

Chapter 16

Cancer, to the person who has it, is an ever-present silent partner. Present, no matter where you are or what you are doing. Present, whether in fact, thought, or suspicion. A simple pimple to anyone else is a possible disaster to the person with cancer. You wonder about how your cancer will be perceived by others. How will it affect your career and your social life. Every spot, every lump, every change must be viewed with a critical eye. I examine myself completely, head to toe, front and back at least once every day, and this accounts for the fact that I have discovered every spot, and discovered them early. I undoubtedly not only have prevented any individual spot from growing large enough to spawn more spots but also have lengthened my own life span. Had I been better informed, perhaps I might have spotted the original primary site and gotten it taken care of before it became as serious as it did. The daily life of the person with cancer is dictated, whether consciously or not, by the disease. You are constantly aware of your own body; you become tuned in to what is going on. My advice to anyone else would always be to trust your own judgment. If you think something is wrong somewhere in your body see your doctor and if he or she tells you nothing is wrong, and you still feel it is, trace it down, see another doctor, but find out what it is that is bothering you. There is a difference between being a hypochondriac and knowing that something is off. I truly believe that people know when something is wrong long before it shows up on any test. However, we are not tuned in enough to our bodies to understand what they are telling us until it can be proven clinically by this test or that scan; unfortunately, many times it is too late by then. If you feel there is something wrong, *do something* until you are satisfied.

You can also live your private and professional lives in spite of the cancer. There is always the temptation of quitting and not fighting as hard, either mentally or physically, or of slacking off the job and feeling sorry for yourself. Even if it is obvious that a person may die, if he or she has put up a good battle and maintained the *quality* of life then he or she is a winner. People who are told they have a terminal disease and quit on the spot are the losers. You have *got* to fight. Fight with everything you can muster. I have found, not only with me but with many cancer patients, that personalities and life styles become more intense after they discover they have cancer than they were before. They work hard, want to accomplish more, and value family and friends more than ever. In my job with Champion I have pushed harder and worked longer hours with more intensity and have produced more than ever. I never want anyone to be able to say that I used cancer as an excuse or a shield to get out of doing anything that was expected of me.

There is a little poem that sums up my feelings, not only as a person battling cancer but also as an athlete and a human being. The poem is written by that most prolific and well-known author, Anonymous, and is entitled "Think."

> If you think you are beaten, you are;
> If you think you dare not, you don't;
> If you like to win, but think you can't,
> It's almost a cinch you won't.

> If you think you'll lose, you're lost;
> For out in the world we find
> Success begins with a fellow's will;
> It's all in the state of the mind.

> If you think you are outclassed, you are;
> You've got to think high to rise;
> You've got to be sure of yourself before
> You can ever win a prize.

Life's battles don't always go
To the stronger or faster man;
But, sooner or later, the man who wins
Is the man who thinks he can.

In my battles with cancer, past, present, and future, when I think I am beaten I will be, but at that time there will have been one hell of a fight put up so that no one will ever be able to say, "He didn't fight it" or "He just gave up without a fight." Yes, there really is a time to give up, but if and when that times comes for me it will be when I am satisfied that I put up the best battle I could.

If you stop and think who really suffers the most when someone dies, it's usually the children. They have never been exposed to death and its associated problems and they have a very difficult time understanding and coping. I remember one incident when I was in the hospital for treatment. It was my birthday and the staff had a birthday cake made for me and they came in and sang "Happy Birthday." Everyone on the floor then knew it was my birthday. A little while later, I got a very beautiful hand-drawn caricature birthday card from a woman and her daughter down the hall. The young girl was a junior high school student and she had drawn the card. She was there visiting her mother, who was dying from lung cancer. I thought how very thoughtful it was of this young girl, who was obviously having a difficult time dealing with her mother's illness, to take the time to draw this beautiful card for someone she didn't even know. It was very touching and I have kept the card ever since. The girl's mother died shortly thereafter and she was torn to pieces. How unfortunate there wasn't someone in her church or school who could have given this girl some help, preferably before the death, in understanding her own feelings and coping with the problems associated with seeing a loved one die. It would be easier if we all understood a little about the process of dying. Not only easier on the person dying but those around him or her too.

After a person dies it is too late to retrace your steps and change your words or actions. You cannot say, "I'm sorry, what I really meant was ————." If we knew a little about what was going on within ourselves and within the person who is dying we could avoid a lot of anguish on both sides, especially the anguish when it is too late and nothing can be done to reverse what has already been said or done. Unfortunately, as Dr. Kubler-Ross has stated and as I have learned firsthand, it is often the older, more established, more respected teachers, doctors, and clergy who are the most resistant to change. They are the ones usually barring the closet doors from being opened and letting the subject of death come out and be debated, argued, studied, examined, and understood by all. I am encouraged that many medical schools are now studying the subject in order to understand what is going on, and that, since the Kubler-Ross studies, studies have been started to learn more from where she left off. We have only scratched the surface of this topic. Even some theological schools have accepted the Kubler-Ross studies and are participating in further studies of this kind. We should know at least the basic fundamentals about the death and dying that will touch each and every one of us several times throughout our lives.

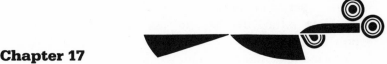

Chapter 17

June 21, 1980: I left for Houston for my ninety-day evaluation and update on how the battle was going. The morning after I arrived I went over to the hospital to begin my testing and as usual everything went very smoothly. After the tests I relaxed a little by walking around the zoo and then jogging about five miles before returning to my room for the evening. Each night I would work about eight hours on the book. I enjoyed this time as it was quiet and peaceful and I could get a lot done without any interruptions. At that time no one had any idea at all that I was writing a book. The following morning Dr. Fredericks gave me a physical examination and then we went over the results of the testing. After studying them a little he just laughed and said, "Mr. Shapiro, whatever it is that you are doing just keep doing it. For some reason that I don't understand you are doing just fine." He went on to tell me I must still be very closely monitored and still have my monthly tests performed but right now everything looked great.

We began discussing interferon. During my most recent previous trip, Dr. Fredericks had mentioned they were doing some work with the drug and I was a prime candidate for its usage. The qualifications to be a prime candidate were really quite simple. If everything else had been tried and failed and there was a measurable, trackable tumor present that could be followed during the course of the interferon treatments, and you were still healthy enough to go through the treatments, you were a prime candidate. I certainly met the first part of the requirements. Everything that had been tried had failed. However, there was not presently any trackable tumor present. I was familiar with the drug, for I had been following its use in the media and the medical journals. It has shown a lot of promise, not only as an anticancer drug but also as an antiviral drug. Dr. Fredericks and I joked about the cost of the drug, which at the time was something like $1.5 billion per ounce—per *ounce*, mind you. I could just see the insurance company getting that bill and saying something like, "Shapiro? Shapiro who? Never heard of him!" Fortunately, the government or the drug company picks up the tab, because no one else could possibly afford to.

Like many of the things the media get their hands on, they hyped interferon way out of proportion and created false hopes all over the place. It wasn't all the media's fault though. They had to get their information from some place and the people at Anderson, and elsewhere, agreed to do the television, newspaper, and magazine interviews and spoke highly and encouragingly about the drug and its prospects. I am sure the reason behind this was to help in future funding for this and associated areas of research. However, the publicity added to the false hopes of thousands of people all over the country. In reality, at that time there were fewer than two hundred people in the entire country who were on the drug or even qualified for it. Dr. Fredericks told me I was still a prime candidate, but that they were having some unexpected problems with it. The side effects they were seeing were more severe than they should have been and they weren't quite sure why. The interferon being used was a natural substance derived from human blood and should have been accepted back into the body with little if any side effects. This was not the case and they didn't know why at the time. He also said they would not administer interferon to me unless an identifiable, measurable, trackable mass was discovered, so that they could follow the use and effects of the drug. In other words, it would be used as a curative-type drug rather than a preventative-type drug.

Every time one of these new drugs gets the publicity that interferon has received, every cancer patient in the world hopes that the long-sought cure has been found and wants to get on the program. However, the reality is that very few people ever get any experimental drug and even fewer have gotten interferon, because of the tremendously high cost and the incredible shortage of the supply of the drug itself. Because the Food and Drug Administration (FDA) has such strict regulations governing the use of experimental drugs, its staff has actually slowed down or retarded the use of some experimentation and has in cases refused to allow some drugs to be used that have shown promise. Admittedly, there must be strict guidelines and rules to follow to prevent unethical, unscrupulous people from taking advantage of and using human beings to test new drugs that have absolutely no business on the market. However, the FDA appears at times to have gone overboard in the other direction.

If there is a viable experimental drug and an institution like M.D.A. believes it can control it and a patient is willing to be a candidate for the drug's use, then I think the choice should be the patient's. If I am dying and there is a drug that shows some promise, provided the proper controls are in effect, then I would be willing to subject myself to the use of the drug. There are two main reasons for this. First is the possibility that the drug just might be the thing to cure me of cancer. Second is the fact that even if it doesn't save my life then at least I would have contributed in a small way to the possible success of the drug and possibly helped to save the lives of others. The important thing, though, is that the choice should be mine; if I am willing to take the risk and I am satisfied with the controls that are in place, and the institution is a reputable one, why shouldn't the choice be mine? Having gone through two experimental drug programs to date with the C-Parvum and another drug called ABPP and considering the many problems I have experienced, I am still, under the proper conditions, willing to partake in future experimental drug programs. There must be controls established and monitored by the FDA, but there must also be a loosening of the laws to permit more experimentation and more research. There must also be an end to placing the research institutions in competition with each other in order to gain funding for their projects. This restricts the sharing of information and encourages the hoarding of it. Perhaps if all the research institutions in the world cooperated, some of the diseases would be cured faster and more efficiently.

It is becoming more and more obvious that surgery is going to be an outdated mode of therapy in the not-too-distant future for most forms of cancer. In theory, at least, a drug that is effective against a particular form of cancer should attack and destroy not only tumor masses but also individual cells that might be floating around with the potential of causing future problems. It makes more sense to me that a drug should be used in conjunction with not against the individual's own immunologic system, which is the basis for all immunotherapy.

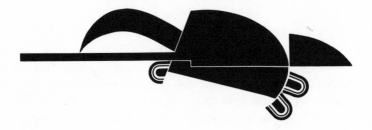

In May of 1981, a very strange thing happened. I'm still not sure if the medical community appreciates its real significance, but it has reinforced one of my own theories as to why I am doing as well as I am. A node appeared directly behind my right ear and was getting larger. I watched it for almost a week and, just as suddenly as it appeared and enlarged, the growth process suddenly stopped. It didn't disappear; it just stayed the same size and didn't change at all. I wasn't sure if it was my imagination or not so I waited to see what happened. Another two weeks passed without any change and I went in to see Dr. Abrams to show it to him and explain that it didn't seem to be getting any bigger; it had just stopped growing for some reason. He didn't like it at all and wanted to remove it as fast as possible. I was about as eager for more surgery as I was to jump off the Empire State Building. After he removed the node we both examined it and there was no doubt at all in either of our minds that this was a malignancy. It was bluish-black in color inside and out. Even the lab, upon preliminary examination, said it was malignant melanoma. I was a little upset about this because I had broken the strange ninety-day cycle I was in and had gone almost a year without a malignancy. This brought me back to reality. I had made the mistake of relaxing a little and I was caught off guard.

When the lab completed the pathological testing on the node, it indicated something that neither Dr. Abrams nor I had ever heard of and the lab people even admitted it was a rarity. All the necessary ingredients were there for that node to be classified as a malignant melanoma, yet it wasn't. It was all necrotic tissue, which means the tissue was dead. All the slides and test results were sent to Dr. Fredericks in Houston and the Anderson lab went over them, reporting the same results. They added that when the tissue was alive it certainly must have been a thriving malignant melanoma. However, what killed it could not be determined.

Several things started crossing my mind at this point. What would have happened had we taken this out when it was still living and growing? The normal thing to do would have been a radical neck dissection; however, since I had already had one, a partial neck dissection would have had to be performed. The reason you can't do two radical neck dissections on one person is that you need at least one of the jugular veins in order to live. That still would have been major surgery though, with some sort of follow-up therapy. The next thing that came to mind was what had happened within my body to kill off this malignancy? What triggered the natural defense mechanisms to start working? How many times had it happened before that we were unaware of? It certainly fits into some of the current thinking about cancer indicating that each of us contracts cancer many thousands of times during our life, perhaps daily, but our body's defense system, the immunologic system, recognizes it and fights it off before it can gain a foothold, and before we are aware of it. I wondered what would have happened in the past had we waited before performing surgery or instituting therapy. Would it have been possible for my own body to have fought off the invading cancer cells? I wondered if it is possible to mentally activate your own body's defense mechanisms. This really started me thinking about the role a person's attitude plays in fighting cancer or any disease.

The really frightening thing about all this is the pattern that seems to be developing over the years. Each time the cancer shows up it seems to be more invasive than the time before, and this makes it more difficult to discover and more difficult for me to fight back to good health. If you want to apply a geometric progression theory to my cancer, and one does indeed seem to be at work here, it gets very frightening indeed. I think that the medical community has missed something here. If the professionals could figure out what is causing my immunologic system to disregard the cancer cells, thereby permitting the cancer to grow and thrive, and then all of a sudden wake up again to what is happening and attack the cancer on its own, as apparently happened with the node, they might have not only the answer to my cancer but also a big step toward the cure of all cancers and all diseases. It almost seems like a short circuit, but a short circuit with a pat- tern. It shorts out only at certain times but is fine at other times. What scares me more than anything else is, if the pattern continues to get more and more invasive, how can I survive continuing bouts?

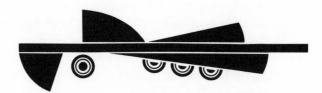

Chapter 19

In May of 1982, I found a spot. I was less concerned about the chance of a malignancy than I was just plain annoyed. For one year I hadn't had any spots or any other cancer-related problems that the doctors or I were aware of. All the test results had been perfect. I went in and showed the new spot to Dr. Abrams and he wasn't impressed with it either, but because of my history and the fact that it was an annoyance he decided to remove it. This spot, now putting the total that we have removed so far in the high forties, was one of the few benign ones.

About three or four weeks after that I started having sporadic stomach pains. I didn't think very much about them until one day they came with such a vengeance that I was completely doubled over. This pain was unlike any I had ever experienced before. I thought it must be ulcers so I went in to see Dr. Johnson. He was a little concerned about it and ordered an upper G.I. to be done immediately. I went downstairs to the lab and we got the test started. After the first three or four pictures were taken, the radiologist said his nurse would finish the procedure and he took off like a bat out of hell. That was my first hint that something was really wrong.

Dr. Johnson had told me he would call me as soon as he had the results, so after the tests I returned home stopping only at a convenience store to pick up a cup of coffee. The office where Dr. Johnson and the lab are located is only about one and a half miles from my house and, even with the one stop I made, it couldn't have taken me more than ten minutes to get home. By the time I arrived, there had already been two calls from Dr. Johnson. He left a message that he was on his way to the hospital and would call me as soon as he got there. When he called a few minutes later he told me the results showed two well-defined tumors in my stomach and that there was indeed an ulcer but it was on one of the tumors. He said he wanted me to have a gastroscopy done first and then go on from there. Before we proceeded though, I wanted to consult with Dr. Abrams.

Lynne was aware that I was going to see Dr. Johnson and she wanted me to call her as soon as I knew anything. I was hesitant to tell her that they had found two tumors in my stomach, but I knew she had already called Dr. Johnson's office twice while I was there. I thought it best that she hear this news from me rather than from Dr. Johnson or one of the nurses in his office. I called her and explained what had happened and I must admit that she took the news very well. I told her that I wanted to consult with Dr. Abrams before making any firm plans.

Dr. Abrams was in surgery all day, but when he returned my call that evening he knew what was going on as Dr. Johnson had caught him between surgeries and had informed him about the events of the day. Dr. Abrams had already consulted with a specialist in gastroenterology and Dr. Fredericks in Houston. Everyone had agreed that the next step had to be a gastroscopy to confirm the results of the upper G.I. The procedure involves the insertion of a thin tube with a scope on the end of it down the throat and into the stomach surveying the stomach and taking the necessary biopsies of the tumors and anything else that seemed suspicious. The procedure was done and the results came back inconclusive. It was decided to repeat the procedure in order to obtain larger and more accurate sections of the tumors. This time there was no question about the results. The tumors were malignant and they were melanoma. The ulcer was on one of the tumors and that was where the pain was originating. I had already started taking something that was blocking the pain and I was able to work and function as normal. As had happened before in my atypical case, it was highly unusual to find a melanoma in the stomach and no one in this area had ever seen one.

All the slides and test results were sent to Dr. Fredericks in Houston and, since I was due back there in less than a week, he said they would take over from that point on. I arrived in Houston on June 20 and started testing on the twenty-first. The results came back as follows: not only were several tumors in my stomach but they also discovered two tumors in my lungs, plus several in my liver. The tumors in my right lung had caused it to partially collapse and Dr. Fredericks said it would totally collapse soon if something wasn't done quickly to prevent it. To say I was shocked is putting it mildly. The only major organs it hadn't hit were my brain and heart. Dr. Fredericks said that he had been expecting this for a long time but not this widespread. He told me that chemotherapy could extend my life expectancy a little bit but not very much. He placed my life expectancy somewhere between three and six months with the probability that it would be closer to three than six. Because of my past experience with chemotherapy and my feelings about it, I refused to take it. As I have mentioned before, I feel that the patient *must* believe in his or her treatment and have full confidence in it in order for it to work. I do not believe in the principle of chemotherapy and could not agree to take it. Even if it did give me a few more months, I would have been miserable and that would have made those around me miserable and would have just prolonged the agony. It would have been quantity time and not quality time. Dr. Fredericks told me of several experimental immunotherapy programs that were getting under way at that time and that I would probably qualify for several of them if I wanted to go that route. Since I was still strong and healthy enough, I would be an ideal candidate for these programs but they would require me to remain in Houston for extended periods of time.

After Dr. Fredericks gave me the results of all the tests and told me what some of my options were, we left it at that for the day and decided to get together again in the morning to see what my decision would be. I needed the time to think about what it was I wanted to do. What was going to be best not only for me but also for my family. I was really shocked at the extent of the cancer. There had been no indications at all that anything was wrong anyplace other than my stomach. I had gone to Houston expecting the problem to be resolved through either surgery or some form of immunotherapy or both. Obviously, surgery was out of the question now because nothing could be done surgically about the liver and it wasn't certain that anything could be done about the lung. Surgery could probably have been of some help in the stomach had that been the only problem area, but with the liver and lungs also involved, surgery was ruled out as an option. By now it was already late in the afternoon and I knew Lynne would be home from school, so I called her and told her what I had learned. I was upset and cried a little but then got control of myself and explained everything. We talked about it for a little while and I told her that I thought I would talk to Dr. Fredericks in the morning and then catch the first flight I could to return home. After talking with Lynne, I called my mother and let her know too. After that I went down to the bar and had a few drinks to just relax and think about what had gone on that day and what my next steps should be. Later that night I called Dr. Abrams, and he was as shocked as I had been. I told him I wanted to get together with him as soon as I got home so that we could discuss my options, if any. I still had a job to do and bills to be paid and didn't think there was any way I could leave my source of income and still support my family.

I went to see Dr. Fredericks in the morning and explained that I didn't think I could just drop everything, leave my job, and be without my source of income while I remained in Houston undergoing therapy. I needed that income so that my family could continue to get along. He said that he understood fully but that if I was going to do something I should do

it soon. He said to call him if I changed my mind. We left it at
that and I returned home thinking it was probably my last
trip to Houston and that I was on my own now. However, I
wasn't quite ready to give in and quit.

After I returned home, Dr. Abrams and I got together to
discuss what had transpired and where we should go from
there. I think he felt worse than I did. I confided in him that
for the first time I thought the fight might be coming to a
close. He wanted to explore with one of the local oncologists a
treatment that some of his patients had undergone with some
success. I agreed to see this particular oncologist. I had heard
several good things about him and I would probably need a
local oncologist on the team now to help with pain control.

I met with this doctor, Dr. Lyons. He had taken the time to
study my case before I arrived. He agreed with everything
that had been done up to that point. He was also of the opinion that chemotherapy could be used to extend my life by several months. I told him in no uncertain terms exactly how I
felt about chemotherapy and how I felt about quantity of life
versus quality of life. Surprisingly, he agreed with everything
I said and we went on to discuss pain control, what approach
we would take and how and when we would begin. I left his
office feeling that at least my last few months alive would be
relatively pain free.

For the first time since I originally contracted cancer, I knew
that I was not only in big trouble but that this time I really was
dying. The cancer was spreading and getting worse. I had developed a little wheezing-type cough that was involuntary
and uncontrollable. This was caused by the tumors in my
lungs. I was also getting tired a lot easier than I ever had
before.

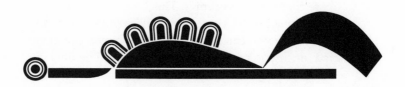

Champion Products, of Rochester, New York, had hired me right out of college. It was my first full-time, permanent job. Champion is a manufacturer of athletic and resale knitwear and sells directly to several different markets. First is the athletic uniform part of the business, which is sold primarily to the high school, junior high school, college, and professional markets. Then there is the resale market, which consists of the college bookstore and school resale areas as well as the retail and recreation markets. The company has been in business over sixty-five years and has always had a family-type atmosphere about it rather than a corporate-type atmosphere. I think that is one of the reasons the officials are so interested in doing the right things for their employees. Rather than try to shrink away from a problem like mine, they have charged full speed ahead in order to help in any way they can. My job with Champion has been to be one of their sales representatives in the state of Michigan. At first I called on nothing but high schools and junior high schools. After a few years of that I was given the responsibility for the colleges and universities in my territory as well. These included such schools as Michigan State, University of Michigan, Eastern Michigan, and Western Michigan. That's where I really found my niche. I not only enjoyed calling on the colleges and universities more than the high schools but I was good at it, too, and therefore my performance continued to improve each year. I did this for nine years before the first signs of melanoma and have been with the company for fifteen years. Fifteen good years too. I would like to think that there are more corporations that would stand by their employees in the way that Champion has stood by me, but I don't think there are. There was always a tremendous amount of freedom in my job as long as the numbers were there (sales volume). This has worked very much in my favor through the years. Regardless of how much you sell or how much you earn in this type of job, you can never be satisfied; once you become satisfied you become negligent and let things slip by and the foundation starts to erode. You must

always be alert for new sources of business and be able to go   **103**
after them. I worked strictly on commission so the more I sold
the more I earned, and if I sold less I earned less. My job gave
me a lot of freedom but it also kept me very active and the
idea of remaining active has always been of prime importance
to me, especially now.

The fears I began having with the advent of the cancer have
been slow in forming but have been very strong and very real
and something I think every breadwinner feels when faced
with the possibility, real or imagined, of losing your job and,
therefore, your means of support. When the basal cell first appeared, I informed Champion as I thought I should. I also
told them it was of little, if any, consequence, and would not
interfere in any way with my job performance. When the second basal cell was discovered, I again informed them in the
same way. However, when we discovered the melanoma, I
told them but I was getting a little uneasy about telling them
too much. I was afraid they might think it was in their best
interests to make some sort of move in order to protect the
business. As things have turned out, my fears have been
eased as they have offered me all the support and assistance I
could have asked, in any and every way possible. I guess
Champion has a great deal of confidence in my judgment and
that of my doctors because, as far as I know, no move to protect their interests was ever taken. They have always maintained that whatever was in my best interest would automat-
ically be in theirs—that keeping me alive and healthy would
be the best thing for them too.

As time went on and I became more involved with other
cancer patients, I began hearing stories about people who
were forced into voluntary retirement or disability or even
lost their jobs altogether because the insurance carrier put un-
due pressure on the company to get rid of the individual with
the very large medical bills. I never really thought Champion
would ever do something like that; however, my medical bills
were getting larger and larger and I was getting more and
more fearful of pressure being placed on the company to do
something to keep the dollar amount of claims down. The

most obvious way to accomplish that with the least inconvenience to the most people would be to eliminate the largest claimant, yours truly. Because of this fear, I worked harder and produced more than I had ever done before. I was not going to give anyone any excuses to get rid of me.

When I was going in for the radical neck dissection, I informed Champion but minimized the seriousness by saying the doctors were sure they could contain it and that the outlook was very optimistic. In other words, I was getting nervous about how much and what I told them. I started telling them what I thought they wanted to hear rather than the straight facts of the situation.

Once my trips to Houston began, I really started holding back information. There were times that I didn't tell anyone within the company I had even gone to Houston. I certainly wasn't going to tell them about the experimental drugs and the possible side effects beforehand. I started telling them edited versions of my experiences, such as the first C-Parvum treatment, afterward, so I could evaluate what and how much I wanted to tell them. I was getting very protective about who knew what and how much. I thought it was ironic that before the cancer I would think nothing of taking a day or two off for no other reason than I wanted to or I was tired and needed the rest. Now, after a night of fun and games with the C-Parvum, when I really could have used a day off to rest, I wouldn't dare take it.

I don't think Champion had ever been faced with someone in my predicament before and I still wasn't willing to take the slightest gamble and let something slip that could cause them to panic and make changes detrimental to me. Most of the people in the front office at the time, with the exception of the new president, had been friends of mine for a good many years, but I still felt my primary obligations were to my family. I knew I had a responsibility to Champion, not legal but moral, and I felt a certain disloyalty about some of my decisions but I just didn't know what to do, and I just couldn't gamble. The stakes were too high for my family and me.

I was becoming more and more protective and was very

careful of what I said to anyone within Champion or anyone who had connections that I thought could become a grapevine back to them, with two exceptions. The other two Champion sales reps in the state and I have always been much closer than just three people working for the same company. I knew that if I ever needed help they would drop whatever they were doing and assist me. If necessary, I am sure they would have covered my territory so that we could have kept my health status from the main office for several months.

When Dr. Fredericks told me for the first time that I was going to die within a relatively short period of time, I again had an internal battle. What should I tell Champion? I could keep the information to myself until the last possible minute or I could tell them right away. Since I wasn't really sure that I believed it myself, I decided to wait until it was a little more obvious, at least to me, that this indeed was true. There was a national sales meeting scheduled for six months from that point and I decided to wait until then to evaluate everything in my own mind and, if I decided to tell them, I could do it in person so that I could defuse any potential problems resulting from my disclosure. I felt that if I did it in person they could see me and see for themselves that I was certainly *not* on my last legs and they in turn would feel confident to leave things as they were. I met with the two other area representatives and told them of the dismal outlook. It's amazing how much better I felt after having told them. They were the first nonmedical people I told. It was very important to me to be able to talk openly and honestly with people I trusted and be able to get their ideas and opinions in return.

If anything happened to me, I wanted one of them to take over my territory and I said I would recommend this to Champion when I told them of the actual situation. I also told them I had not told Lynne about my impending death. Unfortunately, one of them mentioned it to his wife, who inadvertently let it slip at a family get-together a few weeks later. It was several days before I knew this had happened. Lynne had been acting strange and finally blurted out that she knew. I was hurt that she had found out that way; however, I valued the opinions of these two friends too much to cut off our open exchange of ideas.

When the national sales meeting rolled around six months later, I was still not sure of what to do. I felt good, looked good, and had no reason to believe I was dying other than the best doctors in the world had told me I was, but I didn't feel like I was dying nor did I really believe it. I decided to tell at least two people, Harold, the senior vice-president, with whom I have been extremely close since he hired me and put me into part of his territory, and Jerry, the regional manager for my part of the country. I knew I could trust them not to say anything, and I also needed some information on our insurance that I thought they could get for me without revealing why.

I told Harold first. He was very concerned about my welfare and about my fears of telling anyone else within the corporation. He was certain the folks within Champion would not dare turn their backs on me. First, there are laws against discriminating against someone because of having cancer or any other disease and, second, he felt it would destroy the morale and loyalty of the entire company if they did. He stressed that Champion has always taken care of its own and has always prided itself on that fact. This man has meant a lot to me and I trusted him a great deal. I knew he would not lead me astray and I felt much better about things after talking with him. I told Jerry next and he also expressed concern and reiterated that he thought the company would stand by me through everything.

During the week of the sales meeting, the national sales manager came over to me and, without knowledge of recent events, told me that no matter what happens with the cancer I would have my job for as long as I wanted it. He had absolutely no idea what I had told the others and his assurances gave me even more inner security. I can never emphasize how much I appreciated what he did and the tremendous boost it gave me. It also proves a very important point. By assuring an individual with a terminal disease that his job is secure, he will do a better job for the company knowing they are on his side and pulling for him rather than being afraid that if they find out they will find some sort of excuse to get rid of him. I think there is ample evidence to show that a person with a good mental attitude will do better and live longer fighting a disease than will a person with a poor mental attitude. I cannot think of anything that has helped me more than having the complete assurances from Champion that they would be with me and supportive of me in every and any way they possibly could, no matter what. This made me feel more secure but I still felt a tremendous pressure from within to continue producing at a very high level so that there would never be any excuses to get rid of me.

After the disastrous trip to Houston in June of 1982, I knew I owed it to Champion to let them know what was happening. It was obvious that I was dying and it made no sense whatsoever to hide this information from them. It would take two or three months to make the changeover properly and I wanted that to be done as efficiently as possible, with the least amount of disruption, and with the person that I wanted taking over. I called Harold and told him what had transpired and we set it up for me to go to the main office in Rochester to go over the entire situation and decide what the best course of action should be.

I learned that Harold was right when, several years earlier, he had told me Champion takes care of its own. On the day I was to make the most difficult decision of my life, I did it with the help, support, and cooperation of the entire company and, to this day, they continue to stand by me. My fears about repercussions were totally unfounded.

I went to Rochester the night before the meeting was to take place and stayed with Dick and Joan. Dick had been one of the Champion sales reps in Michigan with me but had been transferred back to New York. It was a great night out and, even though my plane was two hours late getting in, we had dinner and then went for a midnight boat ride around the lake they live on. The next day was my birthday, and considering recent events, I couldn't help wondering if it would be my last. Dick and I got to the main office at about 8:30 A.M., so I could have a few minutes to talk with Harold before I started a day full of meetings in order to make some very difficult decisions. My first meeting was with the vice-president of employee relations. He gave me a packet of information that included all my benefits from Champion and my different options, listing the advantages and disadvantages of each. We went over all of them and it became very obvious very quickly that, from a purely logical and unemotional standpoint, my best option was to retire. From an emotional standpoint, it was the last thing I wanted to do, but from a strictly financial standpoint there was a substantial difference between retiring right then or waiting until I physically collapsed and couldn't work anymore. The vice-president of employee relations told me that he and the entire company would stand beside me whatever decision I made and I would have their full support in the future. By the end of the day, I had decided to retire and suggested that they start the paperwork. The decision was tearing me apart. It was not what I wanted to do. I did not feel it was the best thing for me, and I had always said I would never do it. However, it was painfully obvious that it *was* the best thing for my family.

The retirement plan is set up in such a way that your benefits are based upon your previous year's income. If I retired right then and there, I would do so at a much higher level than if I waited until I deteriorated to the point of physically collapsing. At that point my income also would have deteriorated and, therefore, so would my benefits. From a purely selfish standpoint that was fine with me, but I kept asking myself who the benefits really belonged to? It was certainly true that I had earned them and built them up but were they really mine? Whose benefit were they really intended for? From that point of view, the answer was obvious. I couldn't do what was best for me; I had to do what was best for my family. I felt the benefits were there in order to help them reestablish themselves and continue on after me with a minimum amount of financial hardship. I couldn't gamble with something that wasn't mine to gamble with. This, added to the fact that it would give me the opportunity to return to Houston for one last try with one of the experimental drugs

Dr. Fredericks had told me about, made the decision for me. It didn't make it any less wrenching though.

After the meeting with the vice-president of employee relations, Harold and Dick, the president of Champion, took me out to lunch. I was getting to know Dick better now and I must admit that I was impressed with him. I knew he had made several changes in the Champion benefits program specifically with me in mind, and this made me respect him even more—both professionally and personally. After lunch, a birthday cake arrived and I was treated to the honor of having "Happy Birthday" sung to me by the senior vice-president and the president of Champion. I was really touched, especially since I didn't think either of them even knew it was my birthday. The lunch really salvaged my day, since I already was seeing what was the obvious thing to do.

On the plane back home, I did a lot of thinking and concluded that, although I might have just done something I never thought I would do, retire from my job, I was not ready to retire from life. My job now was to concentrate on the fight against cancer and give it my very best effort. That evening I explained everything to Lynne. I don't think she understood it much better than I did, but I explained that, at least for the time being, it was the best decision. In the morning I called Dr. Fredericks and told him what I had done and that I was now available for one of the experimental immunologic programs he had mentioned. I explained that it would take me a few weeks to clear things up but I would then be free to remain in Houston and try one of the drugs. During the next few weeks I saw all of my major college customers I could and introduced Bruce, the man I had chosen as my replacement. Another sales rep was to handle the high school and small college accounts.

On the day I made my decision to retire I asked the vice-president of employee relations what would happen if and when I reached the point that I was able to return to work. He said that it would be a very happy day for him and that I would be placed back on the payroll at once. My job would probably not be in the same territory but I would have employment somewhere within Champion. You cannot believe what a catalyst that has been for me. Knowing I can go back to work if and when I beat this thing is tremendous incentive for me to continue the fight. If and when I recover, Champion should get as much credit as anyone or anything, including hospitals, doctors, and drugs.

Chapter 21

On August 2, 1982, I returned to Houston, and Dr. Fredericks initiated a complete series of tests to see exactly where we stood. My lungs were considerably worse and I was just hours or, at best, a day or two away from one of my lungs collapsing. The liver and stomach weren't much worse than before though, and Dr. Fredericks was glad about that. All things considered, he felt my total condition hadn't changed too drastically from the time I had seen him last. The problem with my lungs had to be taken care of before we proceeded with an immunotherapy program. Dr. Fredericks explained that one of the tumors was growing very rapidly, cutting off the air supply from the bronchi and that once that happened completely the lung would collapse. The only thing to prevent that was to radiate the area and reduce the size of the tumor as much as possible. I felt even stronger about radiation than chemotherapy. He explained this was not a treatment for the disease but a temporary solution to buy time so the immunotherapy could work. He asked me if I would at least talk with the doctors in radiation and let them explain to me what the treatments would consist of, what the side effects would be, and how long they would last. I said I would see the doctors and at least listen to their program and then make up my mind, but my initial reaction was no.

The radiologists examined me and decided what the treatments would consist of and how long they would last. They explained everything to me and I explained my view to them.

I told them I didn't think radiation had any curative benefit for me at all and that the side effects of radiation were too severe and unacceptable for someone in my situation and I felt that rather than prolong my life the radiation would hasten my death. The radiologists felt a ten-day period of radiation on the tumor could prevent cutting off the air supply, thereby preventing the lung from collapsing and giving the immuno-therapy a better chance of success. They didn't think the side effects would be severe and, because of my general good health, I should be able to withstand it very well. They seemed to be telling me what I wanted to hear and I gave my conditional approval on a day-to-day basis only.

The actual radiation treatments were like a very long X ray. The main difference is that once the technician gets you set up for the treatment he or she leaves you in the room and steel doors rumble shut and are sealed, leaving you alone in a dungeonlike room being monitored by T.V. cameras. This is done so that no radiation leaks out of the room and those outside are not exposed. I didn't feel a thing during the treatments but, as the week wore on, I started to get a burning sensation in the area of my chest that was radiated. It felt almost like a sunburn. I also lost all the hair in that area of my chest. After radiation, I returned home for a few days to escape the hospital routine and to assure Jared I was still around. On Sunday we went to brunch with friends and I noticed that as the morning went on my throat was getting sorer and sorer. I thought maybe I was coming down with a cold. By the time I got back to Houston on Monday I could barely swallow. I went to the radiation department and told them what was happening. The doctor in charge of my radiation treatments told me this was the beginning of something he had mentioned before the treatments began. Because my esophagus was between the tumor and the actual radiation beam the treatment would cause a severe sore throat and some difficulty in swallowing. It would continue to worsen for the next three days and then subside, improving each day until it was completely gone. He was right on the money. It happened exactly the way he said it would.

When I arrived in Houston after my trip home, there were four very apparent subcutaneous spots. Dr. Fredericks said these would be good indicators of what, if any, progress was being made. If the spots got smaller or disappeared, it would indicate that the immunotherapy was doing its job. If they grew or didn't change at all, it would indicate that it probably wasn't working at all. After the radiation, I thought the four spots were getting smaller and the doctors agreed. We were all encouraged by this, hoping it was an indication that something good was going on within my body again.

We began the immunotherapy on Tuesday with a drug called ABPP. It stands for 2-amino-5-bromo-6-phenyl-4-pyrimidinol. Now, how's that for a name! Before starting the program under Dr. Alberts, who was in charge of it, I was asked to sign a consent form. I had signed several in the past, but this was the most all-inclusive one I had ever seen. It seemed to protect the hospital and the doctors against everything in the world. I have included a copy of the form. The use of interferon has proven to be totally ineffective in fighting malignant melanoma. However, by using ABPP, it's hoped

---

12.0 CONSENT

NAME _____UNIT NO. _____

I hereby authorize Dr. _____, the attending physician investigator and/or the physician investigator he may designate to administer the treatment: oral administration of ABPP.

1. You are being asked to participate in a phase I study of therapy with an interferon inducing drug named 2-amino-5-bromo-6-phenyl-4-pyrimidinol also known as ABPP. This drug is taken by mouth. It may stimulate the body to produce interferon which is a protein which fights virus infection and may cause tumors to shrink. The main purpose of the study is to find the optimal dose of the drug and to define its toxicity and not to treat your cancer. Anticipated toxicity includes nausea and vomiting and also the possibility of a fall in the white blood cell (infection fighters) or platelet (cells which prevent bleeding) counts. Infection or hemorrhage could result if these fall too low. No other toxicity is expected but it should be emphasized that a phase I study can result in unexpected or unanticipated toxicity. Approximately 30 patients have received the drug thus far and no toxicity has been observed. Interferon was induced in five patients.

2. I have had a description of all the known side effects, discomforts, and **113** risks that may reasonably be expected when receiving this investigational treatment. These effects may include nausea, vomiting, fever, chills, allergic reactions, depression of the blood counts, which may cause an increased susceptibility to hemorrhage and infection.

3. Alternate forms of treatment have been disclosed to me, and it has been made clear to me what possible advantage they might offer me instead of the investigational treatment that I am consenting to receive.

4. I have been given an opportunity to ask questions concerning the therapy involved, and my doctors have clearly been willing to answer any of these inquiries.

5. I have been clearly told that I am able to withdraw my consent and to stop my participation in this therapy at any time and that such withdrawal of consent or discontinuation will not prejudice my physicians against me.

6. Side effects, discomforts and risks that may reasonably be expected to occur are as described above. Other unknown risks, side effects and discomforts may exist. I understand that I cannot expect to receive financial compensation for injury (or death) as a result of participation in the treatment program covered by this consent form and the same is hereby waived.

7. I have been assured that my confidentiality will be preserved and that names of patients will not be revealed in any reports or publications resulting from this study.

With full knowledge of this, I voluntarily consent to receive the above treatment to be received by:

_____
NAME OF PATIENT OR MYSELF

DATE _____TIME: _____

WITNESS: _____SIGNED: _____

PHYSICIAN-INVESTIGATOR   PATIENT OR PERSON
                                     RESPONSIBLE

WITNESS _____RELATIONSHIP _____

I have discussed this project with the subject and/or his authorized representative using the language which is understandable and appropriate. I believe that I have fully informed this patient of the nature of this study and its possible benefits.

_____
PHYSICIAN-INVESTIGATOR

it will force the body to produce its own interferon and fight against the cancer independently. Initially, I was to be given four doses—one each week for four weeks. If it showed some hopeful signs, I would take home enough of the medication to last until I returned again. The first and third days were called pharmacological days. There were to be blood tests at 30 minutes, 60 minutes, 2 hours, 4 hours, 6 hours, 12 hours, 24 hours, and 48 hours. Urine tests would also be performed at the same intervals. Rather than stick me with a needle all those times a heparin lock (a needle that will keep the vein open) was inserted for the duration of the twelve-hour test. The amount of the drug you are given is determined by your height and weight mass. It is given in a pill form. My first treatment was 2,000 milligrams. From there, 4,000 mg, then 8,000 mg, and we maintained the 8,000 level throughout the rest of the program. The only side effects I ever had from ABPP were fatigue and an increased heart rate.

During the four weeks of treatment I kept a close watch on the four remaining subcutaneous spots. By the end of week three, they had completely disappeared. Although the spots had started to disappear before we began the ABPP, Dr. Alberts wanted to continue the drug. It was uncertain what made the spots disappear; however, the test results showed the ABPP raising my interferon levels.

This was the longest period I had ever been away from Lynne and Jared. My mother had come to stay with them and all seemed to be going well. They were apparently getting along well together and that made me feel a little better. It was obvious, though, that Lynne resented my absence. This caused me to resent her resentment and we had several fights over the phone. However, a few hours after each fight I calmed down and tried to understand that it was difficult for her too. She all of a sudden had to take care of everything, including all the things I had always done. She had to do the banking, pay the bills, make sure the lawn was taken care of, and if something went wrong in the house she had to take care of it. She had responsibility for everything with no one to share it.

At the end of the four weeks I was sent home with a supply
of the drug, planning to return to Houston within four to six
weeks for further testing and evaluation. Before I left I under-
went an upper G.I., liver scan, brain scan, and chest X ray. To
everyone's amazement, the test results were as follows: the
stomach was completely void of cancer; there were still two
tumors on the liver, although they showed significant improvement; the brain scan was negative, and the radiation
had been successful on the lungs. Both the tumors on my
lungs were much smaller. I was breathing easier and the little
cough that had driven me bananas had disappeared. Dr. Alberts decided that the best thing to do was nothing at all.
Since I was progressing so well it didn't make sense to change
the course of treatment.

On the trip home I began to settle down. Since May I had
been on an almost nonstop merry-go-round of business, hospitals, tests, retirement, and treatments. Now what would I
do? How the hell would I keep myself busy? I had done a
complete turnaround in my health, from going downhill fast
and knowing death was imminent to the point where my
prognosis was thoroughly up in the air. I could continue to
improve or my condition could suddenly reverse and I could
start going downhill. There was no precedent for my particular case, no way to predict what would happen. I decided to
keep busy through exercise, the final phase of turning over
my territory, and little projects I wanted to complete around
the house. These were all temporary goals meant to take up
time until I got some direction into my life again.

In November I returned to Houston for a week of testing.
The tests indicated I was doing very well. The cancer was still
present in my lungs and liver but showed improvement in
both locations. I was a little disappointed in the results. Since
I was feeling so much better, I was hoping for a clean bill of
health. Dr. Alberts wanted me to continue the ABPP and return in about eight weeks. He said I was the only person in
the world who had taken the ABPP this long and, in fact, I
was the only person in the world currently on ABPP. Dr. Al-

berts couldn't be sure the ABPP was causing my improved condition, but since I continued to improve he had to give more and more credit to the drug. Of course this put me in a rather exclusive club with a limited membership. I have always said I enjoyed my own company but this was a little ridiculous.

Chapter 22

After I returned home with the ABPP, I had a great deal of time on my hands. I started doing all sorts of make-work projects around the house in order to keep myself busy. I became very active in Jared's school in that I was a class parent for his first grade, helping with the parties, chaperoning trips to plays, and generally helping where I could. I was just doing things in order to keep myself busy. After a few months, I realized that that wasn't going to work so I returned to school in order to fill the hours and to take advantage of the time that I had in order to learn about things I had always wanted to study. At Lansing Community College I started out with computers and found that I enjoyed it immensely. I took one course at a time, beginning with the most elementary course I could take and working my way up. Each course I took I enjoyed more than the previous one. I was having a ball. However, I was painfully aware that what I was doing was filling the hours of the day in order to keep myself from going crazy. I wanted to return to work. I missed the satisfaction of being productive, of accomplishing something, of being a contributing member of society.

I returned to Houston in February of 1983 for my checkup and evaluation. On February 15, Dr. Alberts gave me the results of all the tests and scans that I had been taking. There was no sign of any detectable cancer anywhere. My lungs were clean, liver clean, and stomach clean. We were both delighted with this. I'm not sure how or why this happened.

Neither am I sure where the credit should lie. I don't know whether to credit my doctors (and treatments), myself, or divine intervention. I think that a little of the credit belongs in all three places.

I continued taking the ABPP and going to school. In April and June, I returned to Houston for testing with all tests coming out clean. In August my tests again were clean and we discontinued the ABPP. Dr. Abrams said that from that point on, I could have my tests done every three months at home with the results being sent to him.

After six years and all the dire predictions and prognostications, after over forty different surgeries, chemotherapy, radiation therapy, immunotherapy, and being told on three separate occasions that I was going to die in a very short period of time, and after having beaten the odds on all three predictions, I am still alive and kicking, still fighting. I am not sure why, and neither is anyone else. Neither am I sure that I care what the exact reason is because the important thing is that I am still alive. It is up to the experts to make the determination as to why and to apply that knowledge in helping someone else. I think that if anyone had told any of my doctors in June of 1982 that I would be in the state of health that I am in in August of 1983 they would have all agreed it would take quite a miracle for that to happen. I continue to believe that the drugs are only a part of the reason that I am doing as well as I am. In my mind, my attitude that I will not be defeated and my utter contempt for the cancer within me are also significant reasons why I am doing so well.

Several hours after Dr. Alberts and I had reviewed the results of my tests I began feeling frightened. For the past six years I had been living with, planning for, and facing death on a daily basis. I had made sure everything that could be done for my family was done, that everything was in place; there was little, if anything, left to be done except for me to die. I had gotten as much additional insurance as I could, and I had protected Jared and Lynne as best I could in a financial way so that they wouldn't have to worry about how the bills were going to be paid after I was gone. In the spring of 1982, when all my doctors told me that death was between three and six months away, I retired in order to protect my family's financial situation and to give myself one last all-out effort to beat the cancer within me. I felt I owed that not only to my family but also to myself. It would not have been possible for me to have done that while I was working because the only therapies that showed any hope at all required me to be in Houston for several months at a time, with follow-up visits almost monthly. I also felt that I had to be able to give it my utmost mental attention without the daily distractions of work. This was a last-ditch effort that required my complete concentration. I came very close to giving up at that time. I came very, *very* close to just quitting and throwing in the towel, but I didn't. For some strange and inexplicable reason I still felt that I could beat it again. However, I didn't feel that I could gamble with the benefits that would form the basis for my family's support should anything happen to me.

Now that I have spent all this time preparing for, facing, and fighting death, I must start the process in reverse. I must begin to prepare for and return to life. In other words, I must learn how to live again. I'm not quite sure how to do that and that scares me. It has been made abundantly clear that I can return to work for Champion at any time. They have been so incredibly supportive throughout this whole thing that they deserve a great deal of the credit. In truth, without them I could *never* have made it back to this point, it would have been an impossibility. They are truly one of the major reasons I am still alive. They could have easily just made sure that I received everything I had coming to me under the insurance policies that were in effect and left things at that, but they didn't. They went further than just stepping out on a limb for me, they actually stuck their necks out for me and helped in many, many ways. Everyone who is a part of the Champion corporation should be proud and feel secure in knowing that.

There are still several reasons why I must be extremely careful in what I do. When I retired I did so at the top of the ladder with full benefits. The minute I return to work I will be at the bottom and I must start the climb to the top all over

again. If I returned to work I would have to relocate. I couldn't
remain here because that wouldn't be fair to the men who replaced me. However, I could not expect Lynne and Jared to
take that risk, at least for two years or more. Keep in mind
that I am uninsurable and cannot get life insurance of any
kind. That means that I would have to give up the mortgage
insurance I currently have. The consequences of that are that
if I were to die after we had relocated Lynne would be saddled
with a mortgage that she would not have had we remained in
Michigan. If we were to move it would mean leaving the medical team that I have such confidence in, especially Dr. Abrams.
There is a foundation of trust here that I need. I need to know
that these doctors I have been with for so long and have been
through so much with are still with me. I feel a little bit like
the guy who says he is going to retire and the company gives
him a retirement party and then he decides that he is not
going to retire after all. I admit that the situation isn't quite the
same but I can appreciate the way he must have felt.

In February of 1982, I was in Houston for a checkup and got
great reports, no problems at all. In June of 1982, I was in big
trouble with problems virtually everywhere. Now in February of 1983, there is another great report with no problems
anywhere, yet with the odds still stacked incredibly against
me. How can I make a half-way intelligent decision based on
this type of input. I have no assurances that the cancer will
not return tomorrow, next week, or next month. I am well
aware of the fact that in life there are no guarantees at all, you
have to take risks, but you must do so in an intelligent manner with as much input as possible. My initial reaction was
that I wanted to return to work as fast as possible. However, I
knew that would not be the smartest thing to do and that this
was not a time for snap decisions. This is a high-stakes game
and I cannot afford to lose. After I talked it over with my doctors, it was the consensus that the wisest thing for me would
be to remain retired at least until the summer of 1984. The
odds are overwhelming that the cancer will return at some
time but I felt that if I could have three or four years free of it I
could rebuild everything that I would be giving up. However,

I just can't let that happen. Everyone felt I would be the big loser. Everyone thought I would be jumping the gun by returning to work any earlier than that. Some believed that even the summer of 1984 was much too early, considering the odds and the consequences. The big thing at this point was that I could see it happening. I could actually see myself returning to work and regaining the image of myself as a useful, productive, contributing member of society.

It's hard to describe the feeling I had then but it was easily the biggest "turn-on" in my life. I wanted to say "I beat it, I won, I *won*," but I also realized that was a little dangerously premature. I couldn't let myself forget what the odds were and what my actual situation was, not what it appeared to be at that particular moment. I didn't want to be caught off guard again. However, no matter what happens, even if I eventually do die from this, I still believe that I will have won to a certain degree. I was well aware of the very tenuous nature of the situation I was in but, as far as the cancer was concerned, I liked the feelings I was having then one hell of a lot better than the feelings I had had one year previous.

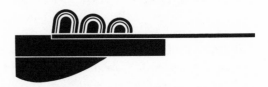

Chapter 23

My trips to Houston were running between $500 and $1,000 each, depending upon the length of time I was there. Except for the two-month stay I was usually there from three to nine days. My medical insurance does not pay for flights or for outpatient room and board while I am there so it was all coming directly out of my pocket and it was getting to be a serious drain. It is a legitimate medical expense and, therefore, a medical deduction for tax purposes and that helped a little. But, like most tax deductions, it first has to come out of your pocket. I have never understood why the insurance company is willing to pay $300 to $400 a day for me to be an inpatient while in Houston but not willing to pay $75 to $100 per day, for room and board, to have me as an outpatient. It doesn't make any sense. However, I have learned that common sense often has no place in the insurance industry. They have been paying for all the work done in the hospital, such as lab work, scans, doctors' fees. Without that I just could not afford to go there as often as I was required to. For the most part the insurance has performed well for me. If I had to do it as an individual I wouldn't have had a chance in hell of getting them to do all that has been done. As an individual you have no leverage and the insurance company couldn't care less about you. However, when you have a company behind you that is willing to stand up for you as Champion has done for me, then the insurance company has to pay a little more attention to things. Without medical insurance you are really in trouble. I feel sorry for people who do not have it and find themselves in a situation like I am in. What can they do? There should be some sort of protection for those people who truly cannot afford to carry medical insurance.

From a personal financial standpoint, cancer can and does cause major problems. Not just financial problems, either, but philosophical problems. For example, when do you stop draining the family's reserves in order to try to survive in the face of impossible odds? Obviously, if there are unlimited reserves, you can continue to try everything and anything regardless of the finances if the will to live is there. However, when, as in my case and in most everyone else's, the reserves are limited and the drain is great, over and above the insurance payments, when is enough enough and who is to make that decision? I am not sure there is an overall answer to that; each family has to make that decision privately. In my case it has not been difficult because I have very definite ideas about it and will not waiver from them. If it were my child or my wife, I would do everything and sacrifice everything in order to know that there was not a stone left unturned in trying to save their lives. I couldn't live with myself if I didn't. I could always make more money and rebuild from the bottom up if necessary. However, I am the major breadwinner in the family, whether from insurance benefits, cash in the bank, or anything else. If I am truly going to die, I think it would be more of a struggle than they could handle to rebuild to the financial level I want for them, and they are going to need those financial reserves to be able to maintain the quality of life that I have worked to obtain. How could I in good conscience spend all our reserves and risk losing everything they would need to live on, just to gamble on treatments that the odds are stacked against? It is true that I built up and earned those benefits, but I am not at all sure in my own mind that they morally belong just to me. If the high-risk treatment worked it would have been a great gamble, but if it didn't and there was nothing left for them, it would make their problems much greater and I just cannot risk that. Therefore, I made the decision a long time ago that, if and when the time came that there was no hope left, I would continue to fight with all my mental and physical powers but would not risk the financial security, whatever it is, of my family and, if that meant no more trips to Houston or anyplace else and I would die, then so be it.

I have several friends who insist that I have sold out, that I have sacrificed myself in order to protect my family and could therefore be hurting my chances for happiness at least and my very survival at most. I don't think there is any doubt that they are right, but what is the alternative? Where is the line that you don't cross where your happiness and survival are not worth risking the future security of your family if and when you die? I don't have an answer for that and I am not sure there is one that would or could apply to all.

I must be very careful even if I do decide to return to work that I do not give up anything I already have in insurance benefits because I can never get them back, unless I want to pay incredibly high rates. Even then, with the higher rates, the insurance companies usually have in the small print at the bottom that there are limited benefits for the first two years. That means they will refund the premiums plus about 6 percent interest. You could do a lot better just putting your money in the bank. The insurance industry has this nifty little computer in Boston that they use to store information about peo-

ple. For instance, every time you fill out an insurance appli-
cation or file an insurance claim, it goes into this computer.
Therefore, someone like me who has cancer and tries to get
more insurance will always be turned down because it is on
file that I have cancer. The most frustrating thing about this
computer though is that they refuse to give you the information they have about you. They claim they will give it to your
doctor but not to you. They really have you over a barrel because if you don't sign their forms they won't pay your claims.
It is really unfair in many instances, too. Suppose a child has
cancer at the age of three and is cured. What happens when
that child is an adult and tries to get life insurance at the age of
thirty? The Boston computer reports that that person had cancer and he or she will most likely be turned down as a high risk
or asked to pay higher premiums. Therefore, I must remain
extremely cautious about what I do because there are things
that I would never be able to regain if I give them up now.

Chapter 24

Based upon my own experiences, whenever I am in a position
of advising other people with cancer on dealing with their
families, I usually tell them to take a close look at the things
I've done and then do the exact opposite. Instead of hiding
things from your family because you question their ability to
handle the disease and/or prognosis, be totally honest with
them. Sooner or later they *must* learn how to deal with it. It
will be easier for them to cope early on with your assistance
and support than on their own after you are gone. If you
should die from your disease, you will have done your family
no favors by protecting them; it will have only made things
worse and more difficult for them to handle. At least, if they
are aware of the actual situation as it happens they can adjust
to things with your help. You will be able to talk with them

and explain how you feel and they will have the chance to express how they feel. Don't underestimate the value of letting them purge themselves of their feelings. It is as important for you to let them talk as it is for them to let you. Both sides have to understand they each have things to work through and it helps tremendously to have those you care about around you and you with them so that each can help to support the other.

Once cancer has been diagnosed, simply putting yourself in your medical team's hands is not enough. You must decide in your own mind that you are going to fight the disease with every weapon, both mental and physical, that you can muster. Medicine, by itself, just is not enough. The will to live must be the most overriding, powerful source of your fight. Ask questions, know what to expect, and be prepared to deal with complications and consequences. These are invaluable assets. Before you expect and demand the very best from your physicians, technicians, and nurses, you must be prepared to give forth your very best. Always keep in mind that you are not only a part of the team, you are the *most important* part. If you have questions, ask them and expect answers and make sure you get them. If you don't understand something, say so, ask for clarification. If you have ideas concerning your case, express them. If you hear about new and different methods of treatment, ask one of your doctors to look into them. If you disagree with something, say so. Don't ever lose sight of the fact that you are in a fight, a *very* high-stakes fight and you need to understand and take advantage of everything that you can. You are not a sheep that is simply following the flock home; you are a person and you need to understand what is happening and how to take advantage of everything you can. Especially, don't ever underestimate the healing or at least delaying powers of your own mind. Too often the scientific community brushes aside the powers of individuals to help cure themselves. The professionals often have the idea that there needs to be a chemical reaction, there needs to be a medicine or an operation or something in order for there to be a cure. Maybe it can't be scientifically proven, but it has been well documented that people *can* effect their own recoveries

both positively and negatively. There are people who have
gotten well when there was no medical reason for them to,
and there have been people who have died when there has
been no medical reason for them to. A lot has to do with the
person's own mental framework. I don't want to imply that all
people who have died from cancer or anything had a bad
mental frame of mind because that is far from the truth. What
I want to say is that people who fight with everything they
can have a better chance of survival than people who have
given up. As I said earlier, there is a time to give up and only
the individual can say when that time is, but until that time
you fight with every available weapon you can use.

Maybe I expect too much from other people, especially
friends and family. After all, I have no choice but to live with
my cancer. For others, it is often easier to ignore it, hide from
it, or pretend it doesn't exist. Perhaps it is a natural defense
mechanism for people to reject cancer and its victim. I know
that all of my family and friends wish me well and yet throughout this whole process I have felt isolated. Again, my advice
to all who find themselves in similar circumstances: avoid doing it my way, alone; it can make things more difficult than
they have to be. To the family and friends of the person with
cancer: not only listen but *hear* what is said and try to understand. If it's too difficult to comprehend everything, say so,
but also say you are willing to try to understand. You will receive an education you will never forget and could never
learn in any classroom. Be honest at least with yourself about
your own anxieties and fears regarding cancer. Sooner or
later, unless there is a monumental breakthrough, cancer will
touch you or someone close to you and you will suddenly be
forced to face the facts—prepared, I hope. Don't be afraid of
your own feelings and fears. The person with cancer has
probably already felt and feared and dealt with them.

My decision to take care of my own funeral arrangements
may not be a popular one with my family. However, by doing
it this way I know things will be done the way I want and I am
assured there will not be any unnecessary and foolish expenses at a time when it is very easy to let your emotions take

over and go overboard. Even if I don't die in the near future, it was still a good move. I want to be in control of as many things that affect myself and my family for as long as I can.

The single most potent weapon I have in my fight against cancer is my son, Jared. It is very difficult for me to accept that he might grow up wondering what kind of a person his father was. Jared is the only child that Lynne and I will ever have and I must admit that we tend to overindulge him at times. But he is truly the best friend I have. I frequently find myself sitting in his room as he sleeps, at two or three in the morning, thinking and wondering about his future. I want to be a part of his future for as long as possible, ensuring that he will grow up to be happy, healthy, secure, and confident. I only hope my cancer won't have a permanent negative effect on him. There are bound to be certain effects though, because a normal childhood usually does not include one of the parents having cancer and even less living the ongoing saga with all the ups and down, surgeries, treatments, and so on that I have had.

I have tried to guarantee his financial future in the event I am not around. I have set up special accounts that will guarantee his education and, to a large degree, a good standard of living for both him and Lynne. I hope he will always remember that no matter what happens, if I die tonight or if I am around for years to come, I will always love him and continue to fight my cancer to ensure he knows that.

My decision to retire had far-reaching implications not only for me but for my family as well. I was not sure what I should tell Jared so that he, a six-year-old boy, would understand. He would obviously notice that I was always home and not going to work anymore. I had learned long ago not to say something I would have to retract later because that just causes more problems. Therefore, I was not about to tell him that I was home now because I was dying. I wasn't sure I believed it, so I couldn't tell him that. I couldn't tell him I was supposed to be a very sick person because to him when you are sick you go to bed for a little while and then you get up and go back to school or out to play. He wouldn't understand it if he saw me doing everything I always did but at the same time said I was sick. I simply decided to tell him I was not working anymore because of the cancer and this would give me a better chance of beating it, plus it would enable me to spend more time with him. He seemed to understand and even like the idea. However, things were not that simple.

One day Jared came in and said he had lost one of his toys and wanted me to take him to the store so he could buy another one to replace it. I told him he would have to learn to be more responsible for his toys and that I was not going to replace the one he had lost. He didn't accept that and kept on about it until I lost my temper and told him his toys were his responsibility and if he couldn't keep track of the ones he had, I was *not* going to replace the ones he lost. With that he told me that he wasn't the only one who couldn't hold on to things, that I couldn't even hold on to my job. That hit me like a ton of bricks. I kept my cool and thought to myself, "Where did that come from?" I realized that Jared didn't understand what was going on and why I was home all the time. Perhaps he didn't like having me home. Maybe I wasn't fulfilling the role model of a father that he wanted and needed. I didn't want my son thinking that I couldn't hold on to a job, but neither could I come out and tell him the reason I wasn't working anymore was because I was supposed to be dying. I just didn't know what to say. I let it go for the moment and the next day I consulted a psychiatrist friend; he gave me two choices. I could bring the subject up again and ask Jared what he had meant or I could wait until he brought it up again. I decided to wait at least for a little while. I didn't have to wait very long.

Ever since Jared was born, I was the one who had night duty and I had always taken him up at night to put him to bed and tuck him in. We always spend a few minutes talking before he goes to sleep, and one night shortly after the above incident we had the following discussion:

Jared: "Dad, do you like working?"

Ken: "When I was working I really enjoyed it and it was very important to me. However, I don't work anymore because I am retired."

Jared: "Well, when you're not tired do you like working?"

Ken: "It's not that I'm tired, I'm *re*tired. That means that I don't work at all. Hopefully, someday I will return to work."

Jared: "Why are you retired?"

Ken: "The reason I'm retired is because of this disease I have that we've told you about called cancer."

Jared: "You can die from that!"

Ken: "Yes, that's possible, but that's also why I go to Texas, to fight this disease and try to prevent that from happening."

Jared: "You better keep going because if you die I'd cry; I don't want you to die, I'd miss you."

Ken: "I don't want to die either, and I am going to do my very best to make sure, if at all possible, that I don't die. I would miss you very much too."

Jared: "What would happen to me if you die?"

Ken: "Mom would still be with you and she would still love you and take care of you."

Jared: "What would happen to me if Mom died while you were in Texas or if you both died?"

Ken: "Jared, if Mom died I wouldn't go to Texas, or if I was already in Texas, I would come right home to be with you. If both Mom and I died, Grandma would be with you or Uncle Jim, but you would always be with someone in our family who would always love you and take care of you. However, I don't want you to worry about something like that because the chances are it would never happen. I do have a very serious disease but I am doing very well right now and I am in no danger of dying soon and neither is Mom. Even if I did die, it would not mean that Mom was going to die."

Jared: "Okay, I love you. See you in the morning."

Ken: "I love you too. Sleep tight."

He then fell asleep, seemingly satisfied with my answers. I certainly hope they gave him some of the assurances he was so obviously looking for.

I still think it causes him some problems because I do not **129** fill the traditional role model of the father going to work everyday. On the other hand, there are times he enjoys having me around. He enjoys having me come to school and do things with his class. I carve the Halloween pumpkin, go to plays, help with parties. He enjoys that. Of course, it's just me and all the mothers and, although I do stick out a little on those occasions, I think Jared enjoys having me there.

Having cancer has taught me a lot about life. My trips to Houston, more than anything else, have demonstrated how easily and how often we misplace our values. How we lose track of the really important things in life.

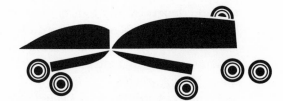

Chapter 25

At M.D.A., you hear many different languages, see people from all parts of the world, all colors, all religions, and all economic and ethnic backgrounds. However, they are all there for the same purpose. Cancer is truly an equal opportunity disease and shows no racial, ethnic, or religious preference. I wish everyone could have the opportunity to just sit and look at and listen to all the people interacting with each other, responding in all ways, verbal and otherwise. There are a few people, like me, who are alone, but not many. It is usually a husband and wife, parent and child, or even entire families. There is no age discrimination either. You see incredible displays of love and caring, as well as resentment and fear. You see frustration and anger, as well as the very quizzical—why me? Why my child? You see small children with no hair from chemotherapy treatments, some even missing a limb or two, yet still remaining cheerful and wanting to play and have fun just like any other kid. You see the very sad and frightening dashes from the hotel to the hospital in the middle of the night, knowing someone has just been notified that a loved one has taken a turn for the worse or perhaps even died. You see people boarding airplanes, so weak they must be carried on board and placed across the seat on a stretcher. That is the world I have learned to live in. I exist in the world as most people see it, but I live in the world of the person with terminal cancer. In Houston, there are many just like me, some better off, some worse, but all in the same boat.

The Texas Medical Center complex is huge and by no means just for cancer patients. Whereas Anderson is exclusively cancer, there are also the Heart Institute right next door, and Children's Hospital, and about six or seven other major hospitals comprising the complex. Ambulances and helicopters arrive and depart twenty-four hours a day, seven days a week. It is truly a medical smorgasbord of maladies. For the most part, the employees are very caring and concerned about the patients' well-being and progress and are certainly conscientious. M.D.A. seems to demand a very high standard among its employees and I haven't been disappointed.

While in Houston I usually stay at a place right across the street from the medical center complex. The place is a hotel, but you must be either a patient or a family member in order to stay there. They have medical personnel on hand and available if needed. All the staff seem to be concerned and want to be helpful. They must enjoy their work because most of them have been there for years.

It is very obvious when patients are new to M.D.A. First, they all look like a lost child, almost overwhelmed by the sheer size of the complex and their unfamiliarity with their surroundings. They are reluctant, in the beginning, to talk about their cancer but soon learn that most people are very understanding of what they are going through and try to make them feel more at ease, both with themselves and with their surroundings. On several occasions I have stopped what I was doing in order to help someone find something or someplace. I am certainly not an expert on M.D.A. but I do know

my way around and if there is something I don't know I know **131**
where I can find out. I like to think that people are more
aware of their own and others' feelings while at M.D.A. After
the first few days or the first few trips you get accustomed to
the workings of the place and feel more comfortable there.
You realize that there is no shame in having cancer and that
others also know what it's like and share your feelings. This
has always reminded me of the part in *Fiddler on the Roof*
where Tevia is talking to God and says, "I know there is no
shame in being poor, but it's no great honor either." That is
what it's like having cancer—there is no shame in it, but it's no
great honor either. The people at the medical center complex
are aware of this also. I don't want to give the impression that
I enjoy my trips to Houston in the sense that one enjoys a vacation; however, I do enjoy the change in values that is dis-
played by the people there. At home I fall into the same traps
as most everyone else: spend too much time on the job, have
too little time for my family, and get too involved with financial matters. I now watch in amazement as adults have temper
tantrums over tennis games and racquetball matches. I am a
very competitive person and I hate to lose; however, I do not
make my living playing tennis or racquetball and know that
winning or losing a game is not going to make any difference
at all in the long run. This is an example of misplaced values.
Being competitive is fine as long as it is kept in perspective.

In Houston, the people around the medical center complex,
especially the patients, seem more people oriented. You don't
hear much about the pressures of the job or about the tennis
game or the golf game. You hear people being concerned
about other people. It can, at times, be terribly gut wrenching, but it is truly what life is all about. From the moment you
walk into M.D.A. you are enveloped by a welcome and caring
atmosphere.

I once overheard the wife of a patient who was obviously
dying confessing to her sister how guilty she felt. She felt
guilty because she wanted to resume her own life and be
freed from the pressures of living with someone dying of cancer. I remained quiet although I wanted to say, "Hey, lady,

don't feel bad. It is normal to want a normal life. Accept your feelings and don't create any more self-doubts than there already are; talk about it and let your feelings out." People on both sides, patients and family, need to be able to talk and unleash their pent-up emotions. However, they need to be able to do this with a complete sense of confidence that what they say will go no further, and that no matter what is said it is all right to say it at that time, no judgments will be made and no recriminations.

The above episode was a turning point for me. I began to give some thought to the conflict of the physician's goals versus the patient's wishes. This thought process has also reinforced my belief in the hospice concept. The ultimate goal in the hospital is the elimination of disease, while the ultimate goal of the hospice is the comfort of the patient. As Kubler-Ross points out, everything the physician learns is geared toward saving and prolonging life. Somewhere, though, the patient's wishes must be considered and become the overriding factor. It is so important in this situation to be up front and let your physician and your family know exactly what your beliefs and wishes are regarding a long, slow death. Should you lapse into a coma or are mentally not able to make decisions all of a sudden, what do you want them to do? Do you want to be kept alive on machines for as long as possible, in the hopes that a miraculous breakthrough occurs and they can cure you? Or do you want the plug pulled? This decision should not be left to the doctors and your family. In sharing your beliefs and wishes with them you are relieving them of the awesome responsibility of making those decisions without knowing your wishes.

Throughout life we strive to learn its true meaning, if any, if possible, attempting to make some sense out of why we are here and trying to attain a certain peace of mind and inner contentment. Just when I began to make some sense out of my life, climbing the ladder to financial security and independence, I got knocked down. I realized that most of the things I thought I knew about life were only superficial with little if any true meaning. After my trips to Houston began, I learned lessons in life that most people are completely unaware of. Very few days pass by that I don't suddenly realize that something that happened yesterday, last week or last month, or the last time I was at M.D.A. has had more of an impact upon my life than it had appeared to have at the time. I might remember the smile a five-year-old child in a wheelchair gave to his mother and suddenly recognize the true love that was being communicated and that, indeed, is what life is really all about.

You might say that I have seen life from three sides, all of them seemingly real but all of them unreal to those who have not experienced them. I have been healthy and completely oblivious of the world of the terminally ill. I have been that terminally ill person, supposedly dying and being able to do nothing about it. And I have been somewhere in the middle, my present position. My world consists of fighting the disease and striving to support my family. It is a confusing position, never knowing what is going to happen next, with the only certainty being uncertainty itself.

Regardless of how comfortable and "at home" you are made to feel, I will never be able to accept certain things as normal, especially the children with cancer. For me the most difficult situation to deal with at M.D.A. is the child and the family of the child with cancer. Every bone in your body screams *Why?* What can one do to help this young life have a chance? I am sure that it must be the same with every disease. Children stricken with disease are much harder to accept than adults.

As you emerge from the elevator on the sixth floor at M.D.A. you turn left and a long hallway leads to the pediatric section. On the corridor wall is a picture of Kermit the Frog, obviously drawn by a child. Kermit is saying, "Welcome to M. D. Anderson Hospital." The picture is in a frame about eight inches wide and about six inches high. On the bottom of the frame is a little plate that reads, "In memory of Lenny, July 26, 1972–May 23, 1982." That sets the tone for the entire pediatric section. In one way it is very depressing to realize that children of all ages suffering serious illnesses have congregated here to die. On the other hand, there is an invigorating, uplifting, loving spirit that is ever present. There are no outward signs of depression in the children or the staff. The children are not there to die; they are there to live, to regain their health and strength, and to return home to normal lives. This will not be the case for all the children, yet that attitude is present in everyone. The children all seem to look out for each other. No one is left alone, everyone is made to feel like part of the group. The entire unit is decorated with bright colors that seem to liven up the place. Most of the kids and many of the staff wear bright yellow T-shirts with rainbows and stars all over them. In other words, everything is geared toward hope and life.

During one of my visits to the pediatric section I inquired about the T-shirts they were wearing. Since it was my business I thought perhaps I could get them a little better price than the one they were paying. When they told me what it was costing them I was sure I could get them a better deal. One of the staff and I sat down and totally redesigned the graphics they were using on the shirt. I decided that, since this was one of the ways in which they raise money for the pediatric section (each child who is admitted to Anderson gets a shirt free and the rest are sold as a fund raiser in order to buy other things for the kids to use and/or play with), I was going to donate the T-shirts to them. In this way everything they made from the sale of the shirts was clear profit. This would give them a lot more to spend on the things they wanted because they wouldn't have to worry about selling x number of shirts in order to pay the bill. I did this for several years, but after I retired I had to stop it because I just couldn't afford it anymore. This is only a very small part of their fund raising but it gave me a great feeling to be able to contribute to something that helped the kids at least a little. If it enabled them to buy a few extra toys, Atari games, books, or whatever, if it helped make the days a little happier for those kids, then it was more than worth it to me. I wish I could have done a lot more.

Each time I am in Houston I try to visit the pediatric floor if I can. During these visits I have gotten to know the woman who runs the pediatric playroom. Her responsibilities include

scheduling activities for the children and she has done a truly
remarkable job. She started a newspaper called *The Sunrise Gazette*, since changed to *The Parade of Stars*. The children write all the articles in the paper, and I have included several that I thought were representative of the pieces written by the kids. Each and every article is *very* important because it allows the kids an opportunity to express what is on their minds. It is very similar to the reason I am writing this book. The woman who ran the playroom when I first went to M.D.A. took a job with the Peace Corps and left for Central America, but the woman who has replaced her is doing an equally outstanding job.

There is also a place for the parents, where they can cook meals and make things as much like home as possible for the youngsters. The children are also required to attend school every weekday they possibly can. A certified teacher from the Houston school district is there who makes sure they do their work and that it is coordinated with the work they are doing in their home school districts.

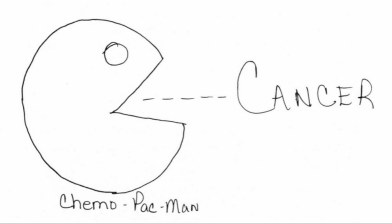

PUBLISHER'S NOTE: The above illustration and the material on the following eight pages have been selected from various issues of *The Sunrise Gazette*, a publication from 6th Floor Pediatrics of M. D. Anderson Hospital and Tumor Institute.

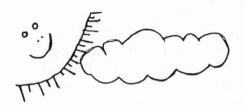

Dear Patients & Parents,

I've Been In And Out Of M.D. Anderson Hospitol For Almost 14 years Now, I Am 19 years of Age. To Those Childern Who Are Now Patients Receiving Radiation And or Chemotherapy I Have only One Bit of And Advice. Never Give Up Your Hope or Will To Live.

My Story Is A Long One, I Will Do My Best Shorten It Sensably. Just After My Fifth (5th) Birthday I Became Quite Ill That Following Spring My Parents Received A Heart Breaking Blow. The Were Told If I Was Not Admitted To M.D. Anderson I Would Have 90 days To Live. I Am Not An Only Child And To Admit Me In This Magnificant Institution They Had To Move The Entire Family Here, You See My Family Is Originally From Indiana.

Though We Were New To Texas We Were Definatly Lucky, We Did Have Relatives In Houston At The Time. I Think That The Fact That Family Branches And Ties Made It Easier For My Parents, But Facing The Death of A Child Cant Be Simple.

All The Troubles And Illness I Have Had I Still Feel I owe My Living To My Parents Tremendous Love And Care, But Also To The Great Staff And Doctors At This Hospitol Along With The Technology & Advances That Are Made Here. All Of You Who Are Going Through What I Did, Never Give Up Hope And Parents Do The Same. By All Means Thats All You Need To Do, The Doctors Know The How To Do The Rest. Listen To Those Doctors They Are Some Of The Best In The Country. If Werent For Their Terrific Knowledge I Wouldnt Be Able To Water Ski, Scuba Dive, Swim or Sick Dive. Please Excuse Any Poor Spelling or Scratch Outs. Remember To Keep Your Chin Up, And Remember I've Been There And Back.

Yours Truly,

Patty Cushman

YOU KNOW WHAT makes <u>ME</u> MaD IS.

Randy Darbone: I hate seeing people smoke in a cancer hospital when smoking causes cancer.

Bubba - The food, cleaning services, no magazines, no weekly B-B-Q's and people who start to like you, like you until they find out you're an amputee.

Rodney Robinson: People with hair

Hiro Nishimura:
needle sticks, staying in the hospital

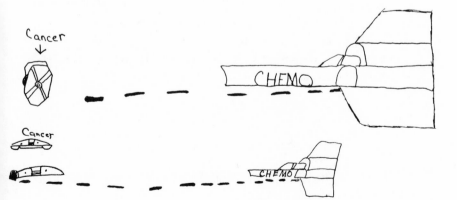

The Day I Got My Subclavian
by Stefanie Guffey   age 11
Houston, TX

Before they came to do my subclavian, I
felt rotten. I was scared because I had
had one before and I knew that they HURT!
They first thing they do is clean off your
skin with betadine and alcohol. Then they
give you some numbing medicine and that
hurts the worst. Then they put in a
little tube called a subclavian. At first
I didn't know what they were doing because
I couldn't feel it but they told me. I
thought "get it over with, get it over with."
Then they put 3 stitches in to hold it in
place (they give you more numbing medicine
for this). I couldn't feel this either.
After that's done they clean it off and
put a clean bandage on. I was relieved
because I knew they were almost finished
Then I started to throw up a little because
I had gotten myself all worked up.

If you have to get a subclavean,
here's my advice: stay still and they'll
get through quicker.

How does it feel to be through with Chemo?

Great, Exciting, Happy, Fabulious, Wonderful and a little sad
because I'll miss my friends. Today is the Tomorrow I dreamed
yesterday. I was told by Doctors in Atlanta my left had to be
amputated first and then Chemo. If I don't I wouldn't live
but 6 months. I wouldn't accept the lost of my leg. A special
friend advised to to go to New York to Sloan Kettering Hospital.
The only differance in the treament was they said Chemo first and
then amputation. I didn't accept this either so, I came to
M.D. Anderson to Dr. Jaffe. Dr. Jaffee also said Chemo then
amputation. He told me the same thing but, for me to let him
think about my case and to finish with the four Chemo treatments from New York and get back in touch with him. I still
didn't have a definite answer. I then went to U.C.A. Medical
Center in Los AngelosCalifornia. (The John Wayne Cancer Clinic)
The Doctor told me Chemo and then amputation of my left leg.
I finish my four treatments from New York so I got back in
touch with Dr. Jaffe. He said that he would go straight Chemo
but, he wanted me to understand this wasn't the normal way this
type of cancer was treated. It was a great risk for me and him.
I said I was willing to try it to save my leg. He gave me
three more treatments of M.T.X. (making seven treatments in all)
Dr. Jaffee made another biopsy. The cancer was gone and I still
Had my leg. Hurrah! Now I've had 33 treatments of follow Chemo
and the cancer is still gone. (These treatments took 18 mos.)
I'll have to come back for check-ups every 6 weeks. You guys
that live close age lucky to have Dr. Jaffe here at M.D. Anderson. He's the Best. He's really cool. Good Luck to all my
friends. Just remember When the going gets tuff, The tuff
get going. I was the first to start on straight Chemo. The
only thing to fear is fear itself. I feel I have won my battle
with cancer and you can too . Hang in there and never give in.
(I know it's tuff). My risk paid off. I want to give thanks
to the following in this order. God, Dr. Jaffe and Reesa, all
the nurses on 6 west and Kelly. I love all of you.

                    Elaine Simpson
                    15 years
                    Atlanta, Georgia

WHY I DID IT
by Johnny Dunn

On Friday, August 6th my central line came out. I had only three more treatments to go. At first I was scared because I thought I would have to have surgery. If the line hadn't come out all the way they would have to do surgery to get it out. They took me from camp to the hospital and took X-rays of my chest and my arm (because maybe it fell down there). They didn't see anything but they said even if some piece were left they couldn't see it without putting dye in.

They put a regular butterfly I.V. in my arm and we left the hospital at 4 o'clock in the morning. We picked up my grandma and flew to Houston. Dr. Jaffe (my doctor) was worried that there was still a piece of my central line left in me but they found out there wasn't.

On Monday Lisa had to put a regular I.V. in my arm so I could get my chemo. She couldn't get it. I was upset and told her I didn't want no more chemo. That was because I have bad veins and I have hard times keeping I.V's and I didn't want them sticking me all the time. The nurses told me I have to have it. I told them they would have one more try. They got one in then pulled it out — I'm not sure why. Maybe it was in a bad place. They said they were going to stick me again so I got up and left.

I went to the Patient and Family Library and read a magazine until I calmed down. I was

continued on.. next page

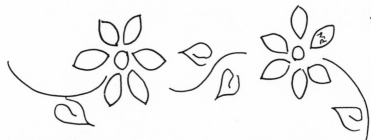

thinking about when I'd have to go back upstairs and get stuck again. I'm sick of getting stuck all the time and especially chemo. I guess I feel this way because I've had it so long.

I finally went back upstairs because I thought my Grandma would be worried and be looking for me. That's when Dr. Jaffee told me I could get another long line or central line for my last 3 treatments. I was real happy and thought it was better than getting stuck each time. Dr. Jaffe told me it was my decision whether to get the long line and take chemo any more. To tell you the truth, I was surprised because I thought he would make me. It was a scary decision to make. I decided to get a central line and finish my treatments. I think it was a wise decision.

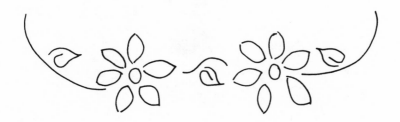

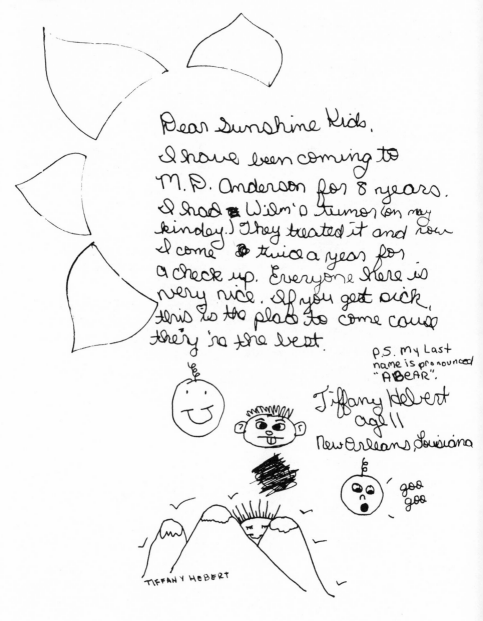

Dear Sunshine Kids,

I have been coming to M.D. Anderson for 8 years. I had a Wilm's tumor (on my kindey.) They treated it and now I come twice a year for a check up. Everyone here is very nice. If you get sick, this is the place to come cause they're the best.

P.S. My Last name is pronounced "ABEAR".

Tiffany Hebert
age 11
New Orleans, Louisiana

goo goo

TIFFANY HEBERT

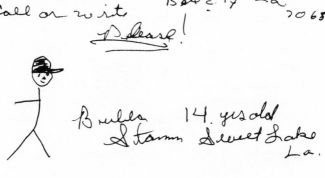

143

Burlea's UPDATE

Dear People,

Doctors say that Osteoe. doesn't come back but it does. My Doctor back home said that the bump was flumiol but they were wrong

I will have surgery tuesday Feb 23, 1982. I thank all of the Doctors over here for saving my life.

I love all of the Doctors.

Burlea Stamm

Ph. 318-598-221   Add. Rt 1 Box 306
                   Bell city La.
Call or writ   70630
      Please!

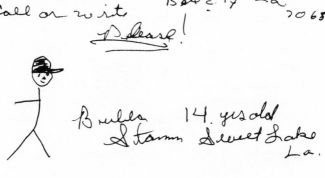

Burlea 14. yrs old
Stamm Sweet Lake
                La.

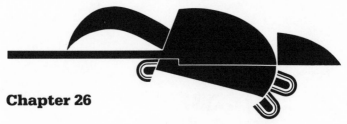

Chapter 26

No matter what has happened to me during my life, I have always tried to keep my sense of humor. I have tried never to take myself so seriously that I could not look back and at least laugh a little at myself or something I was involved in. The fact that I have cancer is serious and nothing to laugh about. However, there have been instances that I can look back at now and at least smile. If we ever let circumstances surrounding us get to the point that we can't laugh a little, then we should just pack it all in and call it quits.

There was an instance during the C-Parvum treatments I can now look back upon and laugh about a little, although I certainly wasn't laughing much at the time. It was one of the times that I just couldn't stand the chills and fever anymore and we called the hospital and informed them I was coming in and to be prepared. Lynne had to stay home to take care of Jared, so I attempted to drive myself. Picture this . . . it was in July and was one of the hottest days of the year, early evening and still in the nineties. Here I was speeding down the road, windows closed, heat on full blast, wearing a heavy-weight hooded sweatshirt, hood up, winter jacket on top of that, sweatpants, two pairs of sweat socks, no shoes, winter gloves on, shivering, teeth chattering a mile a minute, driving down a two-lane, one-way street with my flashers on. It was just my luck that a motorcycle cop was cruising down the road ahead of me, going about ten miles an hour while giving directions to someone in the next lane and thereby blocking me from getting by. Here I was, an aberration, charging right up behind him, honking the horn, and I open the window and start screaming at the top of my lungs for them to get the hell out of my way. For some strange reason the cop moved out of the way and let me go by without a chase or anything.

Most people are aware of the physical destruction that cancer causes but the mental destruction is not as obvious. One of the most powerful weapons we have to fight any disease is our sense of humor. When we can no longer laugh and everything becomes deadly serious, we are well on our way to losing the battle.

Several humorous things have happened with Dr. Abrams, especially in the operating room. That seems to be where we see each other the most. Usually, when a spot is removed it is done through outpatient surgery, so I am awake and watching the entire procedure. During these operations our conversations run through many topics. Sometimes things get pretty silly. Once we started talking about an airplane accident that had occurred recently. Actually, the tailgate stairs on a jetliner had apparently opened or fallen off over southeastern Canada. No one was injured and the plane landed safely. However, we started laughing over some of the funny things that did or could have happened. The stewardesses were apparently serving drinks at the time and the little cart they use rolled down the aisle and out the open stairwell. Suppose you were a farmer plowing your field and out of the heavens comes this little cart filled with all sorts of booze and other drinks and lands right in front of your tractor. It was silly but we all started laughing so hard that Dr. Abrams had to stop for a few minutes before proceeding with the surgery. He was almost crying from laughing so much.

Once during the NCAA basketball tournament, Michigan State University had beaten the University of Pennsylvania the night before by more than a forty-point margin. The nurses were all in green (which is the normal operating room scrub and uniform color anyway, but it is also the Michigan State color) and they had tape on them that said things like Michigan State is Number 1. I was happy about it also because the more games they won the more business it brought to me. I was joking with the nurses and we were all laughing when Dr. Abrams came in looking somber and straight-faced. We continued kidding and joking about the basketball victory

and the game when Dr. Abrams said very quietly, "Does anyone know where I graduated from?" Since I didn't know I
said, "No, where did you graduate from?" He said, "From the
University of Pennsylvania!" I started to get off the operating
table, suggesting that we reschedule this surgery for another
day. Dr. Abrams assured me he would try to overlook the
beating that his alma mater had taken and we went ahead
with the operation. He also said that now he could root for
Michigan State and not feel bad since his team had been eliminated from the tournament.

It is amazing how fast the human mind can work at times.
The next incident is in a way funny but is also a little sad. At
the time it was going on it certainly wasn't funny at all, but
looking back I laugh a little at the incident but not at the
thought process that took place. This occurred in April of
1979 when Michigan State had just won the NCAA basketball
tournament. Because of this victory the bookstores were or-
dering increasingly large quantities of championship T-shirts,
sweatshirts, and other items. We had them on order and all
ready to run if they won and, when they did, we started print-
ing and shipping them air freight as fast as we could. The first
few shipments went fine with no problems. Each order was
larger than the previous one and the quantities that were
being shipped were getting up into the hundreds of cartons at
a time. As fast as they got there they were being ripped off the
shelves; sometimes the store personnel didn't even have time
to get them out of the boxes, people just grabbed them as they
were being put out. After the first few days of this the Teamsters Union went out on strike, which meant that we could
make the shirts and get them from the Champion factories to
the airport in Rochester, New York, on the company's own
trucks and onto the planes going to the Detroit Metro airport,
but from there they couldn't be moved, not even from one terminal to another because the Teamsters controlled everything
that moved by truck and what they didn't control they were
trying to stop any way they could. I figured that the only
thing I could do at that point was to rent a truck and go get
the shipments myself. I had been there several times over the

previous few days checking on other shipments and making sure they were going through smoothly. I had met several of the truck drivers and the people who were working on the docks and found them to be nice reasonable people.

You must keep in mind that I had never driven a truck before and all of a sudden here I am driving this ten-wheeler, which is not huge but is still a large truck, especially when you have never driven one before. The poor people on the highway didn't realize they were in mortal danger just being on the same road with me. I had been listening to the news reports and I had heard that there were picket lines at the airport and especially at the freight terminals, where most of the truck traffic was, and that there had already been some trouble. I thought I could just explain to the people there what the situation was, that I was not trying to break their strike and that I wasn't even a truck driver, that this was a very unique situation with merchandise that was needed immediately and was dated merchandise that would lose its value unless delivered right away. I thought that with this knowledge they would react as normal rational human beings. Not true, they weren't even interested. These were definitely not the same people or even the same type of people I had met before. When I arrived at the freight terminal I was stopped in the driveway by a little yellow Pinto with five men in it. One of them got out of the car, came over to my truck, jumped up on the running board, and asked what I thought I was doing. I explained the situation to him but he wasn't impressed at all. He said that nothing was going in or out of that place as long as they were on strike and that if I was smart I would just turn around and leave. I could see that I was going no place with this guy, and I was not about to just turn around and leave, so I told him to get off my truck and move his car or I would run over it. He wouldn't move so I pushed him off the truck, gunned the engine, swerved around the car, and headed for an open spot near the loading docks where I figured I could park the truck, run into the building, and get help. From there I thought I could get the shipments I was after and head back to East Lansing.

What actually happened was that I got to the parking spot, jumped out of the truck, slammed the door shut, and ran smack into the barrel of a shotgun being held by some guy sitting in the front passenger seat of a camper in the next parking space. The end of the barrel of that gun was less than six inches from the tip of my nose. I realized I wasn't going to outrun that so I stopped, and now he asked me where I thought I was going. Just about then the yellow Pinto pulled up behind the truck, preventing it from moving anywhere. In an instant it dawned on me that this could be *the* ideal situation for me. Here I was, supposedly dying of cancer anyway and facing a long drawn-out and painful death; if I could get this moron who was holding the gun on me to pull the trigger and I died right then, there would be certain advantages that might make it worth it to me. First of all, I would not have a long drawn-out and painful death. Also, it would mean that I would have been killed while on the job and that would mean at least double if not triple indemnity for Lynne and Jared from at least two of the insurance policies that I have. All this thinking occurred in a split second while I was standing there. I said to the guy holding the gun, "Go ahead you ugly —————— ——————, pull the trigger if you have the guts; if not get the hell out of my way because I don't have time to play games with you." At that point, I started to walk away from them. Also, at that exact moment one of the secretaries from the freight building was returning to the building in her car with a package that she had gone to pick up and she had a police escort to get her through the picket line. When my friends saw this they quickly disappeared. From there I got the shipment I was after and started the trip back; however, just to be safe the police gave me an escort for the first ten miles of the trip on the highway to make sure I wasn't being followed. They then turned me loose to terrorize the poor people on the road again.

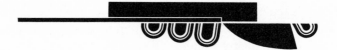

Many people ascribe to the belief that what happens to them in life, whether it be good or bad, is God's will. I have never believed that God is the cause of the tragedies and diseases that afflict humans; instead, I have chosen to believe that we, perhaps not always intentionally, are the root cause for what happens to us. Perhaps we haven't created disease but we have given certain diseases the ideal surroundings in which to proliferate. In the case of cancer, I don't think there is much doubt that our environment and diet are major causes. If people didn't smoke we wouldn't have the major lung cancer outbreaks we have had. If we changed our diets we could cut down on the colon cancers. I prefer to believe in the goodness of God and the ignorance of humans. I am sure that the answers to the diseases we are afflicted with today will be found just as they have been in the past, by persistence in doing the necessary research to find the causes and the cures and not by divine intervention. I am sure that one hundred years from now many of our descendants will look back and say how barbaric we were in the manner in which we treated most types of cancer, by cutting it out. They may wonder why we bombarded cancer patients with radiation and chemicals, often actually restricting the body's own defenses in helping to fight off the disease. I am sure they will look back in amazement at the number of people who died of cancer just as we look back in amazement at the number of people who died from such things as the plague, diphtheria, measles, pneumonia.

I prefer to believe that God has more important things to do than sit around someplace and decide who is going to get what and when, and how it will affect them and their loved ones. In a book I had the opportunity to read recently by a Rabbi Kushner, entitled *When Bad Things Happen to Good People*, I found the author expressing very well what my basic beliefs are. There are points that I definitely disagree with but, in general, he has said that God is not the cause of the tragedies and illnesses of the world. It is not God's will that causes some of the bad things in the world to happen. Some things just happen. There is no reason for it, it just happens, and sometimes it happens to the very people that it shouldn't: the six-month-old baby who is stricken with a disease, the family with small children killed in an accident. These things aren't God's will, they just happen. Where God does step in is by giving us the strength and the courage to fight, to stay alive, to continue on. I could never believe that it was God's will that I contracted cancer because that would also imply that it was God's will that the six-month-old baby contracted cancer or some other disease or that it was God's will that a school bus filled with children was hit by a train. If that were the case it would be a very cruel and vindictive God indeed who would do things such as that, and cruel and vindictive Gods I don't need or want. I don't believe that God is responsible for my personal sufferings nor do I believe that God is responsible for my victories in overcoming the cancer at this point. I do believe that God has given me the strength and the courage to keep on going for as long as I have. I like to believe that God is rooting for me on the sidelines and wants me to overcome, but he is not the cause or the cure of my problems. Religion is a highly personal individualized area and each person should make up his or her own mind in what and how they are going to believe.

There is obviously something working in my favor. The miracles of modern medicine have not cured me but they most certainly have helped me. I have not come this far completely by myself, and I don't believe that it was God's will that I either contracted cancer or that I would do as well against it as I have. However, I do believe that there is a combination of all three at work that is responsible for my survival to this point. All of us have to make our own interpretations of our own or others' situation and come to our own conclusions that make us the most comfortable.

On numerous occasions people have asked me, or inferred, "Aren't you afraid of dying?" And invariably I say, "No, I'm not." Usually they reply with something like, "Man, you've got more guts than I" or just, "That's amazing." However, when you look at it from my point of view why should I be afraid of death? Death is not my enemy, cancer is my enemy, death is actually my friend, my ally. Death will mean an end to the pain and suffering that usually accompany the last stages of cancer. Death is on my side because in the way I have organized this in my mind it means ultimate victory for me over my cancer. It may be hard for people to understand that but I have put this struggle on a very personal basis; it has nothing to do with medicine or with anyone else who has ever had or will ever have cancer. That is for them to contend with on a personal basis and they have had to and will have to deal with their cancers in their own way. For me it is a fight to the finish. If I can kill it with the weapons available to me, I will wind up being the complete victor. If I die from the cancer at this point, I don't think anyone can say that I didn't put up one hell of a fight and that I wasn't at least a partial victor. Perhaps that is not completely logical but it helps me get through each battle and if it does that it doesn't have to be logical. It is the basis of my attitude that it is me against the cancer, a one-on-one fight. As in every contest I have ever participated in I respect my opponent. Cancer is the most formidable opponent I have ever faced. Because it is such a respected opponent I am encouraged to continue fighting for as long as the quality of life is still there. If and when I die from this cancer, death will therefore not have been my enemy but will have become my ally because, when I die, my opponent will die also. As long as I know within me that I have battled to the best of my ability, and for the reasons I have explained earlier, then I will ultimately be a victor in this battle.

Religion can make us more comfortable in dealing with death, but only through comprehensive study of the subject will we ever be able to deal with it intelligently. We can't ignore it and pretend that it only exists for others but not for us. We can't wait until it is staring us in the face to confront it. We should know something about it and decide in our own minds when it is that death is preferable to life. Don't wait until you are faced with making last-minute snap decisions and, especially, don't put it off and onto someone else's back to handle for you. That is not fair to either of you.

Chapter 28

I had gotten off the ABPP in August of 1983 and my tests had been coming out perfect ever since. Things were going along great. Before I stopped taking it I had mentioned to Dr. Alberts a vague pain I had been experiencing on my right side. He examined me and checked over all the test results to make sure that everything was indeed going along as well as we thought. He couldn't find anything wrong at all and since the pain was really no big deal and didn't seem to be getting any worse we just attributed it to a general type pain that comes and goes every once in a while. After I returned home my test results continued to come out great; everyone was amazed at how well things were going, it couldn't have been any better. In January 1984, I went to Rochester, New York, to speak with the executives at Champion about the possibilities of my returning to work. I was getting restless with being retired and I wanted to return to being the useful, productive person that I wanted to be. I knew that it was an enormous risk because the minute I return to work I start all over again at the bottom of the ladder as far as benefits are concerned, and if I died, Jared and Lynne would be the ones to suffer. If I just had a relapse and my benefits were cut to the minimum, we would all suffer. Everyone I spoke to pointed out that I had only been off the drug four months and the medical prognosis was that there would most certainly be a relapse and that this remission was just that, a remission and not a cure. I understood all that but I still wanted to return to work. I spent two days discussing the situation with everyone and just being there reinforced my desire to get back to work with Champion. However, after thinking about it for a few more days and discussing it with my doctors, I decided to wait a little while longer. It was just too big a gamble with something that really didn't belong to me but to my family.

In February 1984, I went to see Dr. Abrams in order to   **153**
schedule my regular three-month testing. In the course of
conversation I mentioned to him that the pain I had told Dr.
Alberts about last August was still there. It felt like a slightly
torn muscle, but I was a little concerned over the fact that it
didn't seem to be going away. Dr. Abrams called the radiologist at the local hospital to ask what tests we might do to
find what was causing the problem. The radiologist recommended that we do a bone scan and a tomogram in addition
to our regular tests. The pain still wasn't getting any worse so
I wasn't concerned that I had a major problem, but whatever it
was I didn't want to let it get out of hand and become a major
problem. I explained this to Dr. Abrams and said that I wanted
a partial CAT scan because all the individual scans that had
been done were telling us what was going on inside the organs
but nothing was telling us what was going on in between the
organs and to me that seemed to be the logical thing to do.
When Dr. Abrams called the radiologist about this he wasn't
too thrilled because he felt that if there was a problem it
would have showed up on one of the other tests and this was
needlessly exposing me to more radiation, not to mention the
cost of the test. I said I still wanted it done regardless of what
the radiologist said.

The test was scheduled for Tuesday, March 27. On Thursday, the twenty-ninth, I called Dr. Abrams to get the results
but he had been out of town for a few days and didn't have
them yet. On Friday, the thirtieth, he called me back with the
results. He told me the test showed a tumor behind the left
kidney about 3 centimeters by 5 centimeters (which is rather
large). This absolutely shocked everyone because what we
were looking for was something on the right side that was
causing the pain I was experiencing. This mass looked like it
was touching the kidney in most of the frames but we couldn't
be certain because in one frame there was a clear separation of
the tumor and the kidney. This whole thing was strange; we
were looking for something on the right side and found something on the left side, and still had no clues as to what was
causing the pain unless it was some sort of referred pain. I felt

more than justified in pushing for this test because if I hadn't we would still be assuming everything was going along great when actually it wasn't. I was amazed that with the exception of the CAT scan all the tests came out perfect just as they had been. The next step was to test the kidney functions, so we scheduled an IVP (intravenous pyelogram), which showed the kidney to be functioning perfectly. The tumor was apparently having no effect at all on that kidney. I called Dr. Alberts in Houston and informed him of what had been happening. He said to send the scans and IVP down to him immediately; as soon as he got them he would go over them with the radiology people at Anderson and get back to me. I sent them the following day Federal Express so that he would have them within twenty-four hours. He got back to me several days later saying that he thought I should get down there as soon as possible so they could follow up with additional tests and some course of action be mapped out.

I met with Dr. Abrams and we discussed the situation in full and I said that in this instance my treatment of choice was going to be surgery because of the size and location of the mass. He agreed with that conclusion and felt that the people at Anderson would be the best qualified to make the final determination and to do the surgery. I was disappointed that he was not going to be doing the surgery but that wasn't his area of expertise and he wanted the people who saw it the most to do it and I agreed with that. I was also keeping Dr. Kenyon fully informed of what was going on and he too was in full agreement that the people at Anderson would be the ones who should see this and make the final determination as to what course of action should be followed, but he was certain that they would also choose the surgery route. I left for Houston that weekend feeling confident that they would opt for the surgery and I would be operated on shortly after I arrived and be home within two to three weeks. I wasn't sure about any follow-up therapy but I would cross that bridge when I came to it.

During the period between the time we found out about the tumor and the time I left for Houston many things oc-

curred to me. The most chilling thing though was that I had
almost returned to work. I had come within an eyelash of deciding to return but had decided at the last minute to wait
awhile longer. Had I returned, it would have been a financial
disaster. In the space of only a few weeks I would have de-
stroyed all that I had strived for during the years that I
had assumed I would die of this disease. It scared the hell
out of me.

The most common question during this period was how
could this have happened. Everyone, including the doctors,
was baffled. Not only were the doctors amazed that there was
something, but the location itself didn't make any sense; melanoma just doesn't go there. If there was going to be a recurrence it would have been a very safe bet that it would be at
one of the spots where it had already been found, not some
other completely off-the-wall place. I suspected that this thing
had been there a lot longer than anyone thought, and it
wouldn't surprise me if it had been there for several years if
not from the very beginning. Lynne was mad as hell at the
fact that this had occurred and had reached the proportions it
had without anyone having any idea at all that it was there.
She questioned all the doctors' knowledge and the validity of
all the tests that I had been taking and questioned what the
good of any of them was since no one or nothing had detected the presence of something that had to have been there
for quite some time in order to have reached the size it was. I
tried explaining to her that neither the doctors nor the tests
were perfect and sometimes these things happen even though
everyone thought everything that could be done was being
done and all tests that should have been taken had been
taken. However, if I want to be honest I must admit that I was
asking myself some of the same questions she was, even
though I knew the answers. It bothered me that there had
never been a complete CAT scan done anywhere. Had that
been done we would at least have had some idea of how long
this thing had been there and which way it was going—was it
growing and getting larger or was it shrinking and disappear-
ing. The only answer I have gotten as to why a CAT scan had

never been done was that there was never any reason. As far as this current tumor was concerned I was totally without any symptoms except for this vague pain I had been experiencing but which still has not been shown to have any connection at all except that I was trying to trace its origin.

I arrived in Houston on Sunday, April 8, and met with Dr. Alberts on Monday the ninth. He started me on another intensive testing program to make sure that the problem was no bigger than we were already aware of. In addition to the regular blood tests and X rays, he ordered a gastroscopy, colonoscopy, ultrasound with a needle biopsy of the tumor, and an upper G.I. series. I had brought with me the CAT scan, liver scan, bone scan, and IVP. After all of that was done we got together again to discuss the results and the total situation. He gave me several different options. Among those he mentioned were chemotherapy, hyperthermia, immunotherapy, and surgery. I eliminated chemotherapy at once on the same grounds that I have in the past. I told Dr. Alberts that in this case my choice of immediate therapy was surgery. He said that was fine with him but he also requested that I speak with the immunotherapy and hyperthermia people too, so that I would know what was available and what they felt they could offer me. In the meantime, he said, he would set up meetings with the surgical people for me so that we could get their ideas and get going on something as soon as possible.

Dr. Alberts told me of an experimental immunologic program they had going there that sounded very promising and he asked me if I would speak with the staff physician in charge of this program. He told me he had already spoken with her about my situation and that she was very interested in speaking with me to see if there was something we could work out to get me on the program. I met with her and she explained that the program involved the use of a new form of gamma interferon, which was supposed to be the purest form of interferon ever produced. She made a very impressive case for it and I must admit that I was very tempted to go with it. She told me they were having excellent results with it against other forms of cancer and that in the lab it showed promising

results against melanoma. She also cautioned me that promising lab results did not always translate to humans. We discussed the two different modalities of surgery and drugs and
the advantages of each. Surgery is a quicker but very limited
solution to a problem. With surgery you go after a specific tumor and remove it without any effect on the cells that might
be growing in another part of the body. Drugs, at least the-
oretically, will destroy not only the main tumor but also any
loose malignant cells that might be harboring in another part
of the body. However, I still wanted to give surgery first crack
at this particular tumor and I told the doctor if that didn't
work I would be back to see her again. She said that from a
medical standpoint either way was a sound decision and that
she would be glad to speak with me again on it if I wanted.

Next I spoke with the hyperthermia people and they also
gave a very impressive presentation on their programs. However, I just wasn't that excited about hyperthermia and I told
them I would keep their proposals in mind, but I was pretty
sure I was going with the surgery and if that didn't work I
would reconsider hyperthermia. I was still convinced in my
own mind that surgery was the correct way to go on this and
perhaps one of these other therapies could be used as a postoperative therapy to make sure nothing else was going on
somewhere else within me that couldn't be detected by the
tests. I was aware that I was an ideal candidate for most of
these programs because I had a measurable tumor that was
easily trackable and yet I was still in excellent general health
and could withstand the rigors of most of these programs
without having to worry about the therapy itself causing
harm. Because I am such a good candidate, I was being cautious and a little wary to make sure everything that was being
said was indeed the truth. Much to the credit of all the physicians that I spoke with, they did not pressure me one way or
the other and were trying to be totally up front with me. They
answered all my questions frankly, honestly, and with pa-
tience and an openness that I greatly appreciated.

I had to wait over the weekend in order to meet with the
surgeons. On Wednesday, April 18, I met with a surgeon who

Dr. Alberts said was one of the foremost in the world in melanoma and if anyone could tell us what the surgical options were, he could. I thought that that was what I was here for, to see the best and get the best opinions I could on the proper course of action. I had a 12:30 P.M. appointment with this doctor and at 2:30 P.M. I finally got to see him. I saw him for about five minutes, during which time he looked at the scans and said he didn't operate in that area, behind the kidney, that it was probably operable, not by him but by the urological people. He sent me down to the urology department and they said under no circumstances would they operate on this mass. It was located in such a way that if they were to do the operation and go in through the flank, as they do, it would shatter the tumor, thereby spreading it all over the place. In the doctor's exact words, "If I did that surgery I guarantee you the cancer would spread at the very least throughout the entire abdominal cavity and I just won't do that." They then sent me back to the first surgeon who said he just didn't think it was in my best interest to have this surgery. He went on to say that what scared him the most was not what he saw on the scans but what he didn't see. He went on to explain that, from his experience, once he got in there he would find that the tumor was attached to the retroperitoneal wall and had spread throughout the muscles in my back causing him to have to remove not only the tumor and the kidney but such a large portion of the diaphragm and the muscle in my back that it almost couldn't be done. Even at that, he said, if he went ahead with the surgery anyway, he didn't feel he could get any more than 75 percent of the tumor, leaving me in exactly the same position I was in in the first place. To say the least, I was stunned. I had been positive this thing was going to be operable and here I was being told by several top-notch surgeons that not only wasn't it operable but it wouldn't be in my best interests to even attempt it.

After that I returned to Dr. Alberts and explained what had happened; he too called the first surgeon and discussed it with him. I told him that I was disturbed not only at the deci-

sion but also by the way the decision was made. The urological surgeon explained why he thought it inadvisable to
operate and it seemed to make sense to me. However, I didn't
like it that the first surgeon made this decision that has such
a huge impact on me after spending less than five minutes
on the examination and consultation. Dr. Alberts said that
he was a little surprised this was inoperable, too, but these
surgeons see these things every day and they have learned
to manage their time efficiently. If this is what they think
then most probably that is the way it is. We decided to get together in the morning to decide what course to follow now.

I was bothered all night about not only the decision but also
the way the decision was made. I met with Dr. Alberts in the
morning and we discussed the entire situation again and he
said that it was always an option for me to seek an outside
second opinion on the surgery and I should keep that in mind.
We went on to discuss the other options still open to me and
we decided that the gamma interferon program seemed like
the best for me at this time. He said he would set up the ap-
pointments for me and I agreed, but I also said I was going to
keep the surgical option open. I explained that I had too
much at stake to let the decision be made not on the basis of
what is shown in the scans but what is not shown, and base
everything on the experience of the surgeon, no matter how
good that surgeon is or how big his or her reputation is. If
there is one chance in a million that they are wrong then I
should take it. After all, what's the worst thing that could happen? They could open me up, take a look, and say, "Yes, that's
the correct decision," and close me back up again, but at least
I would have the peace of mind of knowing for sure that was
the correct decision and not base everything on speculation. I
can't stand the thought that upon my death and an autopsy
someone might say, "Gee, you know that could have been
taken out had they just tried." If the scans confirmed what
the surgeon suspected, I would have been able to accept the
diagnosis, but without that confirmation there has to be some
risks taken by someone at some time.

I met again with the physician in charge of the gamma interferon program and told her what had transpired with the
surgeons. She went over in detail what the program she was
offering entailed. It would require me to remain in Houston
for a minimum of six weeks getting daily shots. At the end of
that period another ultrasound would be taken and a determination would be made based upon the size of the tumor at
that point as to whether or not the drug was having any effect. If it was I would have to remain in Houston for an inde-
terminate period of time and continue to get the daily shots
for as long as the drug seemed to be having an effect on the
tumor. The main side effects, once we got into the program
after the first few days, were supposed to be those of a mild
case of the flu. The first few days were supposed to be the
worst but once past them it was supposed to be just a mild
case of the flu, low-grade fever, mild chills, a little achiness,
and some fatigue. I gave my tentative approval to start the
program but based it on the condition that I would remain
there for the six weeks and at that time they would release the
drug to my doctors in Lansing for me to continue with the
program. They said they would try but the FDA had not given
approval for this drug to be released yet and since they were
the only place in the country that was using it their hands
were tied. They said they would try their best though and we
left it at that. I explained my experiences with C-Parvum to
the doctor and told her I had heard the mild-flu routine before, and I was nervous about it. I felt better that I would be
right there in case anything went wrong and the doctor assured me that no matter what time of the day it was there
would *always* be someone around who could handle any
problems that came up and that she was always available as
well. She told me they would do their very best to control the
side effects, and if they got out of hand they would get me off
the program; they had no intentions of making anyone suffer
unnecessarily. I also said that before getting started on this
program I wanted to return home for a little while since I had
already been away for more than two weeks, and since I was

going to be gone for at least another six weeks I wanted a little time to spend with my family before getting started. They weren't wild about this idea but they agreed.

While home I met with Dr. Abrams and Dr. Kenyon to discuss the situation and let them know what had transpired and to get their input on it. Dr. Abrams was a little surprised that the tumor was inoperable but he said that they do see these things every day and if they determined it was inoperable they were probably correct. However, he also agreed that I should keep the surgical option open. Dr. Kenyon was a little more than surprised. He felt they had made a mistake and the tumor was operable. I told both doctors I was going to give this drug a shot and if it didn't work I would look at the surgical route again. While home I also had the chance to be with Jared and go to a few of his soccer matches and see the start of his softball season. We talked about the fact that I would be gone for awhile but that I would be talking with him at least four or five times a week and I would be coming home again without any doubts about it at all. I also explained the program to Lynne and what it entailed and she was in agreement with it, at least at the time I left for Houston again. On the day I left, I took Jared to school and gave him a hug and a kiss as I always do when he leaves for school, but this time I started to cry. I had been through this too many times before and I didn't want to leave him again. It was a very emotional time for me. After I regained control, we spoke for a few minutes and he went in to school. I drove home after that and after I got in the house I just sat and cried for a few minutes as the whole thing was starting to get to me. It occurred to me that there was nothing forcing me to return to Houston and I could change my decision at any time before I got on that plane. However, upon thinking about it, I realized that was a very short-sighted approach and that I was doing the correct thing in the long run. Everyone needs to just let go every once in awhile and although it is extremely rare for me to do that it was good for me. All the pent-up emotions just seemed to flow out. After that I got my bags and left for the airport.

I arrived back in Houston late in the afternoon of Tuesday, May 1. On the second, I spent the day taking the base line tests that would mark the starting point of the program, and at five o'clock that afternoon I met with the doctor in order to go over the results and prepare to start the program the following morning. However, she said that the radiologist, in comparing the results of the ultrasound test taken that morning with those of the one taken two weeks previously, felt there had been very significant shrinkage in the size of the tumor in that time period. She said she had serious doubts about that but wanted to get together with the radiologist and go over the test results with him the following day and we should get together again then to go over the results and make a decision on the drug program. If it were true it would mean that I was starting to go into another spontaneous remission and they didn't want to do anything at all to interfere with that. We set up an appointment for 4:00 P.M. the following day. My spirits skyrocketed at this news. I was trying to control myself and not let my hopes get unrealistic. After all, the doctor did say she had serious doubts about the results and that sometimes there is a mistake in comparing the tests and she wanted to make certain of the results.

We met at four o'clock the following day and she said she had met with the radiologist and gone over the results with him and he was standing by his determination that there had been significant shrinkage in the size of the tumor. However, she still had serious doubts about the results and the two of them decided that the best thing to do would be to take another CAT scan and compare it to the one that had been taken in Lansing in March, when we originally discovered this problem. The CAT scan was scheduled for Monday at 7:30 P.M., but I was also put on a waiting list in case they had any cancellations and could get me in sooner. They called that night saying they could get me in if I got right over there, which I did without any delay. I was really flying high at this point and I was already thinking about returning home the following week without having to undergo any treatments at all. We would finally have the proof that my body was doing the good work all along and this last test was going to prove it to be true.

I called the doctor first thing in the morning to let her know the scan had been done the previous night. We set up an appointment at four that afternoon so we could review the results of the test and determine what we were going to do. I was sure the test would show a reduction in the size of the tumor; after all, two ultrasounds and the radiologist reviewing them not once but twice and standing by his decision that there was indeed significant reduction just couldn't be wrong. When we got together that afternoon the doctor told me the test showed no change at all, either way, and she thought we should proceed with the treatment as planned. I don't want to say I was crushed because I had kept telling myself to be prepared for the worst, and the doctor had kept telling me she thought the results were wrong, but I was greatly disappointed. I guess I was a little angry, too, because I had been told the ultrasound was going to be the test of choice to determine whether or not the drug was having any effect upon the tumor. I didn't understand why all of a sudden the ultrasound was not the test of choice and we couldn't rely on its accuracy. On the other hand, I couldn't very well complain about their trying to be as thorough and complete as possible in order to get the true results and not be taking any chances. None of the tests is infallible and sometimes using one test to check another test is a good thing to do, especially when the results of the first test are in doubt. It was like fighting emotions with facts. The facts were that there was no change and, no matter how disappointed I was, the facts were still the facts. We decided to go ahead with the program and I was told to report at 7:30 A.M. Monday to get started.

Saturday and Sunday were free days and I needed them. I needed to get my state of mind back to the point where I could get behind this treatment program and give it the best chance I could. On Saturday I just relaxed and rested. On Sunday I spent the day with Mary and Harry. It was the perfect way to spend the last day before therapy began because it gave me a chance to get away from the medical side of things and spend some time with friends in a relaxed friendly atmosphere and just regroup myself so I would be ready to get started.

The first day of the program is a pharmacological day, which means that blood tests had to be done at specific intervals during the day, so I was told to meet the doctor at 7:30 A.M. in order to get started with the blood tests and then get my first shot. I was there on time, the doctor wasn't. The nurses got me started with the blood tests and put a heparin lock in place so they wouldn't have to stick me with another needle each time they took blood. The doctor finally showed up at 9:15 A.M. and I was angry. I felt that, if I was asked to be someplace at a specific time in order to get started on a program that was as important as this one was to me, the least I could expect was that the doctor be there on time too. I was probably a little on edge about getting started but I also believed I had a valid point. I was having a few doubts about whether or not this program would be for me if this was the way things were going to be.

I received my first shot at 9:30 A.M. After about an hour and a half I started to get mild chills that lasted approximately fifteen minutes. After that my temperature started to go up and reached 102 degrees at its highest point during that first day. That was the way it went during most of the day. Mild chills, followed by an increase in temperature. The worst part was the achiness; that was a little tough at times but overall I thought I did very well. A little difficult at times but not unbearable. It was an emotionally draining day though because I was afraid of it turning into another C-Parvum–type program and indeed it did seem to be similar in the type and order of the side effects—the chills and then the fever with achiness thrown in for good measure, and I was going to avoid that at all costs. Fortunately, it was all on a much lower scale than the C-Parvum, at least for that day. The fever never reached the same heights nor were the chills and achiness as bad. The doctor came in and she also said I had done very well that first day. By five in the afternoon I was feeling a great deal better and I was allowed to return to my room for the night.

Starting with day 2, unless it was a pharmacological day or there were some other tests that were to be run, I was to report in every day at about 8:30 A.M. to get my shot, wait an hour for my vital signs to be checked, and then I could leave for the day. Day 2 was easy. I reported in, got my shot, waited for the hour, got my vital signs taken, and then left and had a very pleasant day. During the day I had no real side effects at all, just some mild fatigue. I even went out to dinner that night, which turned out to be a mistake because in the middle of dinner I started getting side effects, such as chills. However, even this wasn't very bad and I just finished dinner and went back to my room and relaxed for the rest of the night. I really didn't experience any other side effects that day or night. I felt that if that was the way things were going to be I was going to be able to get through this program relatively easily. However, I wasn't to get off that easily. Beginning on day 3 the side effects started getting worse not better. I was told that after the first few days things would get much better and after the first week I would only have mild side effects at best. As usual, with me it didn't happen that way. The side effects were increasing not decreasing after the first few days and they never stopped increasing. Even after the first week they just kept getting worse and worse. The shots were supposed to alternate from left arm to right arm to left hip to right hip and back to left arm. Whenever I was given a shot in the hip I developed a rash from my hip down to my ankle that lasted a few days. We had to stop giving shots in the hip because of this and we alternated between arms. I started developing headaches that were getting more and more severe and got to the point of being unbearable. I couldn't stand any noise or light, and the pain was vicious. The achiness was getting worse and, combined with the chills, also became almost unbearable. My feeling was that I was getting more severe side effects each day we continued, and it was becoming another C-Parvum.

The doctor was trying her best to minimize the side effects. She would give me one pain killer after the other trying to find something that would work on the headaches. Then I couldn't sleep, so she gave me something for that; she was really doing the best she could to make things easier for me. I can't blame her because after the first day when I had to wait for her she was very attentive and concerned. I was losing weight and that alarmed everyone except me. I couldn't eat because the side effects were so bad. I was more concerned about the other things because once they were taken care of I would feel more like eating and once I was eating properly again I would start to regain the weight. Finally, after the eighteenth day, when I started throwing up and could barely make it across the street, I told them that I didn't think this program was going to be for me. Unless they could do something to take care of the headaches and the other side effects that I was experiencing I didn't think I could continue with the gamma interferon. It was getting to be that I was trying to survive against the drug, with the cancer being secondary. There were several other people on the drug at the same time that I was and we would see each other every day and talk. I would ask them what type of side effects they were having and none of them seemed to be experiencing what I was. I met with the doctor again and told her I had decided to take myself off the program because the side effects seemed to be increasing rather than decreasing and after eighteen days I didn't think that was right. She told me she thought that I was making a mistake and she didn't agree with my decision but she went along with it. I told her that if she developed something that would lessen the side effects a little I might consider taking the drug again. Since it did seem to be showing some signs of hope in certain forms of cancer, I wanted to keep that option open if possible.

I met with Dr. Alberts and told him what had happened and that I was going to return home and get some rest and consider what I wanted to do from there. He agreed with me but said not to let too much time go by because it was important that we do something. I said I would stay in touch. I left not knowing what I was going to do. My first reaction was to try to look into the surgical option again because I still felt the decision that this was not operable was wrong. I wasn't angry, because I think the doctors involved were making a decision based on their best medical judgment and I can't fault them for that. It was just my gut reaction that the decision was wrong and I at least wanted to look into the possibility of someone going in and confirming the diagnosis of inoperability or, if it was operable, performing the surgery. I wanted to give myself the best chance possible and I felt strongly that I had to look into this option.

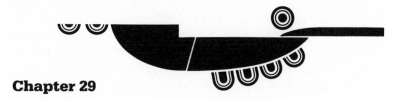

Chapter 29

There was no way in the world that I could just get on a plane and return home in the condition I was in so I took the next two days and just rested, slept, got out and walked around in the sunshine, and just did a lot of nothing. I returned home on Wednesday, May 30. For the first few days I rested some more and enjoyed being home and off the treatments. After that I got started on doing something about the problem I was having. I met with Dr. Kenyon and he wanted me to see a surgeon at Ford Hospital in Detroit. He was sure that surgery was the right course to follow and wanted me to speak with this surgeon. I met with Dr. Abrams and told him what I was planning on doing and he said that there was no harm in it and to see what the surgeon had to say.

I met with Dr. Diaz on June 12. We had a very long, frank, open conversation and covered a lot of ground. I was impressed with him and he was with me. He told me that when he originally agreed to see me as a favor to another doctor he was certain that it would be a very short visit with no resulting surgery because anyone with melanoma where I have it definitely also has it in the liver and probably in the lungs as well and any surgery at that point would be useless and cruel to put the patient through and he would not do it. When he saw me walk in he didn't think I was the right person because before him was an obviously healthy person who could not have metastic melanoma. When he confirmed that I was who I was indeed supposed to be, he was fascinated and we went over my entire history of melanoma and what had been done. I explained to him that this tumor had been declared inoperable by other experts and why they thought so. I also said that I couldn't go on the basis of someone's experience without actual test results confirming the diagnosis, no matter who the surgeon or how great his or her experience. I went on to explain that I couldn't understand why someone didn't just go in there and confirm the diagnosis. If it was right I have lost nothing and have gained the peace of mind that I had tried everything. If it was wrong I have gotten rid of that tumor and given my body and any future drug programs a better chance of success. Much to my surprise, he agreed and said that he thought it would be a good move to go in and look around at this point. Furthermore, from the scans and ultrasounds that I had brought with me, he thought that it was operable. It would be major, major surgery but it was possible. I asked him if he would call Dr. Abrams and Dr. Alberts and discuss it with them and he agreed. I said I would also discuss it with them and from what I learned from their reactions plus my own thoughts about it I would make my decision and would call him the following week. Actually, I had already made my decision without telling him. He had given me a sense of confidence that he could indeed do this surgery and that he knew what he was talking about. I had decided in my own mind that unless Dr. Abrams and Dr. Alberts could give me a reason not to do it I would go ahead.

I discussed the entire situation with both Dr. Abrams and Dr. Alberts and they said they were impressed with Dr. Diaz' presentation of the situation and his confidence that he could remove the tumor successfully. Neither of them had any reason to tell me not to go with the surgery and therefore they confirmed what I had already decided to do. I called Dr. Diaz the following week and we scheduled the surgery for Wednesday, June 27. I entered the hospital on Monday, June 25, in order for them to perform certain tests that they wanted to do and to get started on nonabsorbable antibiotics. This was **169** being done just in case they had to actually enter the bowel. The antibiotics would neutralize the bacteria that would otherwise be a major problem if the bowel were opened either by accident or intentionally during the surgery. They did an arteriogram and another ultrasound, chest X rays, and several more blood tests. I was taken off all solid foods and was allowed only clear liquids for the two days prior to the surgery.

During this entire process I had been discussing all the issues with Lynne and she was in agreement with everything that was being done. I had been keeping my mother somewhat informed of the situation as she was there when I returned from Houston and there was no way I could avoid it. She had come while I was in Houston in order to help Lynne while she and Jared were both still in school, and she was indeed a big help and we appreciated it. She returned to New York after I returned from Houston but wanted to come back for the surgery and I agreed to that. However, the same old problems were cropping up between my wife and my mother, so I was a little apprehensive about having the two of them together during the surgery and going at each other. However, this time my cousin from Kentucky came up for the operation and she was placed in the position of being the peacekeeper. Several friends had come up from Lansing to be with Lynne during the surgery and they too helped keep the peace.

The night before the surgery, Dr. Diaz came in and told me that they had discovered another mass just behind the prostate and that he was certain it was involved with the melanoma and we should reconsider everything at this point. I asked him if he thought it was malignant and he said he was pretty sure it was but that the only way to be certain was to get a biopsy and have the lab make that determination. He went on to tell me that most surgeons would cancel the operation at this point but he thought mine was a unique situation and he would do whatever I wanted him to do. I said that at this point I wanted to take one thing at a time and that I wanted to go ahead with the surgery and while they were doing that they could get the biopsy of the other mass and I would worry about that later on. It was my feeling that I was again presented with a situation where we could not tell how long this mass had been there and whether it was getting bigger or smaller or was completely dormant. I felt that for me, in this particular situation, it would be best to proceed and get rid of the major mass and relieve my body's defenses from worrying about that one. Dr. Diaz agreed and we proceeded as scheduled. After he left, Lynne and a friend had come in just to say hello and good-bye quickly as visiting hours were long over. I told them about what had transpired but I don't think either one of them understood at the time what I was saying or the implications of this new development. I also told them not to tell my mother because at this point the last thing I needed was for her to get more upset and get everyone else upset about this. I didn't think she could handle it all at that time as she was very upset about the original surgery without having to worry about something else. I also informed Dr. Diaz that this new situation was to be discussed with no one other than me. I was making the decisions and going on my own best instincts and just didn't need any outside interference at this point and especially not right after major surgery. There just wasn't enough time now to inform everyone and after surgery I was going to be in no condition to be going over anything new at all. I felt that this course of action was going to be the best for me at this time.

The surgery was scheduled for eight o'clock the following morning. After everyone had left for the night, the nurses came in and gave me an enema to make sure that I was completely cleaned out before the surgery. They came in again at about six in the morning to give me a mild sedative and something else to make sure that I was on my way out before they took me down for surgery. Everyone came in to wish me luck right before I was taken down and we all crowded into the same elevator going down. When they could go no farther I said good-bye to everyone and that I would see them later that day. Usually I can remember being rolled into the operating room and being switched over to the operating table, but this time I can't remember even getting into the operating room. I

can remember talking to Dr. Diaz and some of the surgical
nurses outside the operating room, but then they gave me
something and that is the last thing I remember. The surgery
took a little over six hours and I withstood it very well. I was
sent back to my room afterward rather than intensive care because I was doing so well. The one thing I had been very clear
about with Dr. Diaz was that I wanted to be kept as pain free
as possible after this surgery. I had been told that there would
be a good amount of pain involved and I wanted to avoid as
much of it as I could. After I was back in my room and awake,
a pain killer was the first thing I asked for because I was in
great pain. I must admit that the staff was right there on the
spot whenever I needed them. They gave me shots every four
hours with something else in between that would enhance
the original shot. Pain is not one of my most favorite things
and if they could keep me free of it, especially those first few
days when it was supposed to be the worst, that is what I
wanted them to do.

The following day when I was more awake and aware of
everything that was going on, Dr. Diaz came in before any
visitors were allowed and we discussed the surgery and how
it went and what he found. He told me that he was very surprised the surgery went as well as it did, that the tumor was
not attached to the retroperitoneal wall as the surgeons in
Houston had feared, and that it was easier to get to than even
he had suspected. It was still major surgery but he didn't have
to remove as much of the diaphragm or as much muscle and
tissue as he had feared he would. In short, it went great,
much better than we had any right to have hoped for. Hind-
sight is always twenty-twenty but this apparently was a case
where too much emphasis was placed on the tests and personal experience and not enough on taking a chance and my
personal feelings. I still refuse to blame anyone though, because the doctors in Houston were using their best medical
judgment on this, and most often they would be correct. I
can't blame them for that. However, the bad part was that the
biopsy taken of the mass behind the prostate showed that it
was indeed malignant melanoma, plus he found four small

(about 3 mm) spots that "looked clearly like melanoma metas-
tases." The large mass we had been aware of, but the four
smaller ones were a surprise to both of us. We discussed the
situation and Dr. Diaz said that it was highly possible there
were many, many more of these small spots throughout my
body. I felt they were so small that if my immunological system would click on again it could easily destroy them. Because of this I was glad that we had done the surgery in order
to get rid of the bigger mass. I felt that this was going to give
my body more of a fighting chance.

We discussed what should be done about this new large
mass and it really presents a dilemma. My first question was
whether or not it could be removed surgically. Dr. Diaz answered in two ways, first from a strictly technical basis. Yes, it
was possible to do; however, the price was going to be very
high from a real life point of view. He explained that it would
again require major surgery that would cause them to have to
find other routes for the bowels and urine, cause total impo-
tency, and in the long run really not have that great a chance
of getting rid of the cancer, just this one tumor. I objected on
many grounds and ruled out that surgery immediately. The
price was just too high. Two things I had said I would never
do: retire, which I eventually did anyway, and allow myself to
be taken apart piece by piece and this would have been a big
step toward that without any assurances that it would do any
good while I was being assured that it would definitely and
permanently disfigure me. In my mind it would disfigure me
not only physically but, more importantly, mentally as well.
As it is I look like I was put together with a sewing machine
but this new surgery would be just too high a price for me to
pay. As I have maintained throughout everything, there is a
quality of life that must be maintained and the only judge of
what that quality level is, is the person involved.

We next started to discuss alternatives; the first one he mentioned was chemotherapy and I eliminated that right away.
Next we talked about radiation and that did seem to have
some possibilities, although I was under the impression that
radiation in that area has terrible side effects. I did agree to at

least speak with the radiation people there at the hospital. I   **173**
said that any therapies would probably be done in Houston
because that is where I have the most confidence in the staff
but I also wanted to keep an open mind. Dr. Diaz said he
would have the radiation people come up to see me in a few
days and we left it like that for the time being. It seems there
is no end to this constant cycle of ups and downs; every little
bit of success seems to be flattened out with more obstacles.
However, I am determined to continue the fight for as long as
I think it is worth fighting. The radiation people came in several days later and presented their thoughts on this therapy
and how it would apply to me, but I just wasn't impressed
enough to go ahead with it. I am sure that any therapies I
agree to will be done in Houston because, as I have already
stated, I want to give myself the best shot at it I can and I believe the folks at M.D.A. are the ones who can offer it to me.

Dr. Diaz had said he was going to keep me in the hospital at
least ten days after the surgery but I said that I would be going
home one week after the surgery and I was right. On July 4,
Lynne and a friend of ours came to pick me up and take me
home. Lynne and my mother had been kept apart so there
were no fights between the two of them. Lynne had gone
home after the surgery in order to be with Jared while my
mother and cousin remained in Detroit for several days. Then
they too returned to their homes. I was glad that there were
no major uprisings during that period. It was something I
could easily do without. I had explained exactly what was
happening and what was going to happen to Jared so that he
didn't feel left out by not knowing what was going on or getting confused when he heard others talking about it. I wanted
to assure him that I was going to come through this surgery
fine and that I would be coming home to him again. Lynne
had brought him in on Sunday after the surgery to see me
and, although it was a very brief visit, I think it did both him
and me a great deal of good to be able to see each other.

The recuperation period from this surgery was going to be
more difficult and would last longer than past recoveries simply because more pain was involved due to the area of the

surgery and more was taken out than during any other surgery that I have had. I could see that I was tiring easily and that I required naps in the afternoon in order to make it through the day. However, I could also see that each day I was getting a little stronger and felt a little better than the previous day. I got out and exercised each day and started doing things, such as going to Jared's softball games and his swimming meets almost as soon as I got home. I can't stand just sitting or lying around doing nothing. I was thinking a great deal about what it was that I wanted to do but was coming up with nothing. Dr. Alberts called me one day to see how everything was going and I told him about the surgery and what had been found. We discussed it and I told him he would be receiving the postoperative report shortly from Dr. Diaz and after that I wanted to go to Houston and discuss the situation. He said he was glad everything had gone well and that as soon as he got the report he would let me know and we would make plans for my return to Anderson. However, the one thing that has kept popping up in my mind is that sooner or later doing nothing is going to be better than doing something and perhaps this was that time. It seems to be a medically sound, viable option at this time. I would be gambling that my immunological system would click on again and fight the cancer on its own. It has done it in the past and it could do it again. I think the best thing for me to do at this point is to listen to what all my options are and then take a little time to consider what it is I really want and go from there.

Obviously, this story is not going to be over until it is over, until I either die or live my life cancer free. Because of that, there is no better place to end this book than right here. I am again faced with a situation I have encountered so many times before. It highlights the point that people with cancer live with total uncertainty and have to continuously be on their toes and aware of what is going on within themselves. The struggle against cancer is not an easy one and each person has to take control of his or her own situation and make some very difficult decisions. You can't just sit back and let the decisions be made for you. You have much too much at stake to let other people be making these decisions. I don't know what it is I am going to do at this point but you can bet that whatever it is I will make the choice, and I will consider it very carefully. I will look into what is best for me, the individual, what the odds are for and against, and will decide when the time is right to go against the odds.

Currently I am forty-two years old and have had cancer for the past seven years. Jared is now eight years old, which means that for all but one year of his life his father has had cancer and he has been brought up in this atmosphere. He has known nothing else and I hope and pray that there has not been too much damage caused because of it and that some good will come out of this. I know he worries about me dying and I try to answer all his questions honestly yet in such a way that it does not appear that I will die shortly. Lynne and I have been married for sixteen years now and seven of them have been hell for her. Perhaps fate has dealt me a bad hand due to this cancer, but it has been downright cruel to her. There is no one less well equipped to handle something like this than Lynne. Not that anyone is really well equipped to handle it, but Lynne has had and continues to have a very difficult time dealing with it. I feel sorry for her but I don't know what to do to make things easier for her. Currently she is having a very difficult time, and very understandably too, dealing with the fact that there are at least five tumors that we are aware of and are doing nothing about, at least temporarily, while we try to figure out what they are doing and are likely to do in the near future. I have explained the reasons why I am doing what I am doing but she wants assurances of success and of course no one can give them. I remain retired and I will probably return to school again. I had to drop out of my last class because I had to leave for Houston for six weeks, at the least, for treatments, and since the course was only twelve weeks long to begin with I had no other choice. I can't say what tomorrow is going to bring. Usually it's as much of a surprise to me as it is to everyone else. However, I can say this: things must change, the status quo is totally unaccept-able to me, I need more. I'm really not sure in my own mind what that means but I do know something is missing, there is a void that has to be filled. I think what I have to do is to re-establish myself to myself. I'm not sure how to do that yet, but sooner or later I will. With luck, it will be sooner.

My major hope for this book is that someone somewhere will read it and feel a little better knowing that there are others who are going through this too and understand the mental and physical pain he or she is having. I hope people will learn from my experiences. If ever you or someone close to you contracts a terminal illness, or any illness, I hope you will learn to face it with them and share it with them. Deal with the situation as it is and not as you would like it to be. Listen to what you are told by the doctors whether you are the patient or the family, but don't hesitate to ask questions and demand answers. If you don't understand something, say so and make sure that you understand everything that is happening. Know what is going on, and not only be a part of it, make sure you, as the patient, are the major part of it.

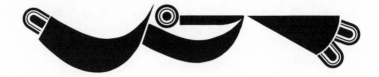